SPINAL CORD INJURY
A Guide for Patient and Family

Contributing authors:

Catherine W. Britell, M.D.
Juan Fonseca, M.D.
M. Elizabeth Bayless, M.M.S.C., R.D.

Illustrations by Samuel R. McFarland

This book was prepared under the auspices of the
Paralyzed Veterans of America.

SPINAL CORD INJURY

A GUIDE FOR PATIENT AND FAMILY

Lynn Phillips
Mark N. Ozer, M.D.
Peter Axelson, M.S.M.E.
Howard Chizeck, Ph.D.

Raven Press ☙ New York

Raven Press, 1185 Avenue of the Americas, New York, New York 10036

Made in the United States of America

Library of Congress Cataloging-in-Publication Data

Spinal cord injury.

  Bibliography: p.
  Includes index.
  1. Spinal cord—Wounds and injuries—Patients—
Care.   2. Spinal cord—Wounds and injuries—Psychological
aspects.   3. Spinal cord—Wounds and injuries—Social
aspects.   I. Phillips, Lynn. [DNLM: 1. Spinal Cord
Injuries—popular works.   WL 400 S75775]
RD594.3.S6684   1987   617'.482044   84-42866
ISBN 0-88167-274-2
ISBN 0-88167-275-0 (soft)

9   8   7   6   5   4   3   2   1

*For the men and women of PVA
and all others with spinal cord injuries*

Preface

Each of us who wrote this book has had considerable personal experience with disability: either as one who became spinal cord–injured, as a family member whose role was not well defined, or as a caregiver in the weeks and months after our "patients" sustained their disabilities. Each of us sees spinal cord injury from a different perspective, and each has information about spinal cord injury that we believe is useful to share with you.

If you are newly injured, we want to help you avoid unnecessary difficulties and heartaches. If you are a relative of someone who just became disabled, we want to offer to you in one book all the information that it took us years to uncover.

If you have had a spinal cord injury, it is our expectation that this book will provide you with information and familiarize you with resources that would routinely otherwise not be accessible to you. Those of us who are physicians want to provide you with the basic medical information that we wish all our patients had available so that they could participate actively and fully in their rehabilitation process and in promoting good health thereafter.

Our overall objective is to present a basic and comprehensive guidebook to spinal cord injury such that, even if your questions are not answered in this book, the references listed will help you locate those answers.

Lynn Phillips
Mark N. Ozer, M.D.
Peter Axelson, M.S.M.E.
Howard Chizeck, Ph.D.
Catherine W. Britell, M.D.
Juan Fonseca, M.D.
M. Elizabeth Bayless, M.M.S.C., R.D.

Acknowledgments

A multidisciplinary book such as this is dependent upon the cooperation, contributions, and critical analysis of many people. My coauthors and illustrator, all of whom agreed to write their chapters without pay as a gift to the Paralyzed Veterans of America (PVA) Spinal Cord Research Foundation, deserve special thanks and commendation. Mark N. Ozer, Peter Axelson, Juan Fonseca, Howard Chizeck, M. Elizabeth Bayless, Catherine Britell, and Sam McFarland devoted much personal time and effort to this project.

A number of friends and colleagues willingly read the manuscript or parts of it and contributed ideas for changes or additions to it. While the authors accept full responsibility for any errors that may exist, I would like to thank the following people who reviewed the manuscript before publication: M. John Anderson, Arlene Battis, Chad Crowley, Ann Grandjean, Marolyn Halverson, Stephen Little, Sue Mahler, Pat Mann, George Murray, Angelo Nicosia, Ruth Hall Phillips, Gail Price, Diana Schneider, Labe Scheinberg, and Roberta Trieschmann.

I also would like to thank R. Jack Powell, Executive Director of PVA, for his encouragement and support during the preparation of the manuscript.

The unsung heroes of this book, however, are the PVA Research Department staff and our part-time assistants who, despite the frenetic pace of everyday activity at PVA, gave devoted attention to preparation of this book. Tom Stripling, Priscilla Craig, Deberah Moses, Jeanne Ann McVey, Ann Barker, and Denise Stevens all played pivotal roles in what became a much larger task than we ever had imagined.

All royalties from the sale of this book have been assigned to the PVA Spinal Cord Research Foundation to encourage research that will alleviate the condition of spinal cord injury in the future.

Lynn Phillips

Foreword

When I was paralyzed four decades ago, medical knowledge of spinal cord injury was still rudimentary. Nevertheless, I was among the lucky ones who eventually regained use of both legs and one arm, although my right arm remains paralyzed. We learn a lot about ourselves, those of us who have experienced this trauma. We learn that courage is mental as well as physical, and we come to understand that courage means overcoming fear, not just being fearless.

To suddenly find oneself paralyzed is a devastating experience, not only for the individual but for family and friends as well. During the first few hours and days after injury, the only people the patient can turn to for information and guidance, for answers to questions, and for reassurance about the future are the medical personnel. These people are completely engrossed in the immediate problem of your survival and maintaining and restoring as much function as possible to the damaged cord.

Spinal Cord Injury: A Guide for Patient and Family is a valuable resource that will fill the inevitable gaps left by the medical team. This book responds in lay terms to the many medical, social, and psychological questions that will crowd your mind in the days, weeks, and months following your injury.

The medical chapter will help you understand the physical implications of your injury and what you can do to minimize the complications to your general health. Other chapters will help you adjust to your new life, provide information about daily living, and suggest ways in which you can adapt your lifestyle to maximize the physical capabilities that still remain. There is a wealth of information in the appendixes that will help you to locate the services that are available to you in both the private and public sectors.

I found the chapters by Peter Axelson particularly enlightening. During a decade of living with paralysis, Axelson has found that there is not much that he cannot accomplish if he is willing to find ways to get around his disability. Today, 10 years after his accident, he does most of the things he did before—only now he does them differently. And for those activities that he can no longer manage, he has substituted an alternative which he now finds equally, and in some cases more, rewarding.

Before World War II practically nothing was known about spinal cord injury, and few people survived the ordeal. Casualties of that war increased the number of spinal cord–injured persons dramatically, and with that increase came the urgent need to understand the chain reaction that is triggered by injury to the spinal cord.

During the early years of my own injury, my body was overwhelmed by infection, my temperature rose to an incredible 108.7 degrees, and only the removal of one kidney brought the situation under control. Later, my life was threatened again by obstruction of the lung by blood clots, and medications available at that time proved ineffective. Consequently, I became a "guinea pig" for a new drug. No one knew what, if anything, the drug would do, but streptomycin saved my life, as it has saved countless lives since.

Although a cure for the problems that result from a spinal cord injury is still a long way off, knowledge of the various components of the puzzle grows daily, and we now dare to hope that solutions will be found. Many dedicated people are working in spinal cord research trying to make that hope a reality. Until that day, this book will provide you with information you need to live a useful and satisfying life and maintain good physical condition, so that whatever medical advances the future holds, you will be ready to take advantage of them.

United States Senate   *Senator Bob Dole*
June 1987

Contents

Contributors

Peter Axelson, *5858 Empire Grade, Santa Cruz, CA 95060*

Elizabeth Bayless, *Spinal Cord Injury Service, Veterans Administration Medical Center, 1201 Broad Rock Road, Richmond, VA 23249*

Catherine W. Britell, *Spinal Cord Injury Service, Veterans Administration Medical Center, Seattle, WA 98108*

Howard Chizeck, *Case Western Reserve University, 611 Crawford Hall, Cleveland, OH 44106*

Senator Robert Dole, *Hart Senate Office Building, Room 151, Washington, D.C. 20510*

Juan Fonseca, *19040 Wentworth Drive, Hialeah, FL 33015*

Mark N. Ozer, *Spinal Cord Injury Service, Veterans Administration Medical Center, 1201 Broad Rock Road, Richmond, VA 23249*

Lynn Phillips, *507–1540 29th Street N.W., Calgary, Alberta T2N 4M1, Canada*

CHAPTER 1

Dealing with a New Injury

Lynn Phillips and Peter Axelson

A spinal cord injury is not "just" a physical disability. It also can profoundly affect the way we view ourselves and others around us. Society today places great emphasis on youth, physical prowess, beauty, and overall appearance. When we or a member of our family is permanently disabled, we are confronted not only by the reality of disability but also by a lifetime's misperceptions and prejudices about disability.

Spinal cord injury generally occurs as a result of a single, traumatic insult to the cord. It could be the result of a car accident, a sports injury, or a gunshot wound that occurs as a result of being in the wrong place at the wrong time. In almost all instances, spinal cord injury occurs to someone who only an instant before was a perfectly healthy, active individual.

Within a split second, life can be altered drastically. And, just as each person reacts differently to crisis, we each have our own way of reacting to and dealing with a spinal cord injury.

A common initial reaction to spinal cord injury is refusal to accept the severity of the injury. Many patients and their families steadfastly maintain from the outset that "This is a person who is going to walk out of this facility."

Such a reaction is common and quite normal and often with good reason. Many of us have read accounts in the popular press of "miraculous" cures or of people who have been told

1

by their physicians that they would never be able to walk again only to leave the hospital unassisted. What may not have stayed in our memories is that the injury was badly broken hips or vertebrae in the back, not a compressed spinal cord. Sometimes the spinal cord is simply bruised as opposed to being crushed or severed, but these cases usually are identified early by surgeons and the injured individual and the family are so informed.

Refusal to accept the seriousness of the situation may be due as much to externally influenced expectations as it is to an inherent need of human beings to avoid unacceptable realities. Furthermore, it is important to hope that things will get better because hope is a positive motivational force. Nevertheless, physicians and other professionals who work with newly injured patients and families can be especially helpful by explaining in clear, simple terms what the chances for any kind of motor or sensory recovery are and what factors lead them to believe that the disability may be permanent.

GETTING THE FACTS

For many people, the first step toward adjustment to spinal cord injury is obtaining information about the full extent of the injury and its implications. A realistic picture from your physician about the exact nature of your injury, as well as the physician's expectations for the extent of functional recovery, are important pieces of information for making decisions about how to accommodate your needs and interests to the inevitable constraints.

Traditionally, physicians have had difficulty being the "bearers of bad news" to patients and family members. A serious, ongoing debate in the medical profession concerns the ethical question of how much to tell a patient and when. For traumatic injuries like SCI, as well as for terminally ill patients or for persons with chronic diseases, like multiple sclerosis, many physicians believe that the patient's interests are best served by withholding negative details until a direct question is asked. This viewpoint holds that the physician's role is to "protect" the patient and family from as much unnecessary pain as possible.

The other side of the argument (and the position taken in this book) is that you have a *right* to know as much about your condition as possible and that only with full, informed knowledge of your condition can you make intelligent decisions about your life.

The ethical debate on this question continues. In the meantime, if you want complete information about your condition and a physician's informed, honest opinion about the prognosis you may have to ask specific questions to get that information.

What questions does one ask? The first question probably should be, what is the *level* of injury? Chapter 2 discusses levels of injury and the functional recovery that can be expected at each one. It also discusses which body functions, such as bladder or bowel control, will be affected at each level of injury.

The next question should be, is this a *complete* or *incomplete* injury? A complete injury means that no signals can be transmitted from the part of the cord above the injury to the area below, or vice versa, and that there is no feeling and no movement below the level of injury. Incomplete injuries, on the other hand, imply that some "messages" are getting through.

When injuries are incomplete some function may be recovered below the level of injury, but the degree of recovery is difficult to predict. Nevertheless, information about the extent of injury is necessary for reevaluating your priorities and reacting to the limitations that may be imposed.

REACTION TO DISABILITY

Another frequent reaction to spinal cord injury is anger. Sometimes that anger is directed against oneself, particularly if the injury occurred as a result of personal error or care-lessness. In other instances the anger is directed at the person who is perceived as being the cause of the injury, such as a drunk driver. In many cases the injury may not have been preventable and there is no one to blame which is itself a frustration. Consequently, anger is directed toward hospital staff, society at large, or even those who may have been in a similar situation but escaped permanent injury.

Anger is a natural outlet used by human beings to cope with loss of control and frightening or threatening situations. Other common responses to spinal cord injury are depression, anx-iety, or any number of other emotions. How you respond de-pends on how you generally have responded to stressful sit-uations rather than on any "typical" pattern of response.

Most rehabilitation professionals recognize that anger and other emotions are "natural" reactions to what is an unex-pected, wholly unwanted change in your life. Consequently, psychologists, social workers, and other trained professionals are available at most medical facilities to provide individual and family counseling and to give you and your family psy-chological tools for coping with a severe disability.

Many facilities also conduct patient and family education classes that teach self-care techniques, introduce you to po-tentially awkward social situations, and provide basic infor-mation about how the body responds to an injury to the spinal cord. Information sessions such as these can be helpful as you begin to reconstruct your life.

During the initial hospitalization and in-hospital rehabili-tation phase, patients and their families have easy access to knowledgeable support people among the hospital staff. Re-habilitation, however, is a process that begins in the hospital but continues long after you go home. For many people with spinal cord injuries, the return home is a particularly vulner-able time. Although in a familiar setting, the fact that you cannot get around your own home without the assistance of other people, a wheelchair, or crutches can be difficult to accept. The daily routine of therapy sessions, patient education classes, and self-care activities on a regimented hospital schedule no longer exists when you are at home. The supportive world of staff who are familiar with SCI and other patients and families with similar situations no longer provides an informal support network. Once home, you and your family may feel totally alone and without help or support. Combined with the difficulty of reestablishing your preinjury routine and lifestyle, the adjustment period after hospital treatment can be even more traumatic than the days and weeks immediately following injury.

The transition will be easier if you acknowledge that there may be difficulties and if you plan beforehand to address potential problems. Some rehabilitation facilities have established peer counseling programs to aid in the transition from patient to active member of the community once again. Peer counseling matches a newly injured individual with a person in the community who sustained a similar injury and has successfully reentered community living. The role of a peer counselor is to provide support and assistance in "learning the ropes" of adjusting to life after a spinal cord injury. Independent living centers, which are centers run by and for individuals with disabilities, also can serve as an excellent resource during the transition period.

Some Veterans Administration Spinal Cord Injury Centers have a program called Hospital-Based Home Care (HBHC) to assist you in the transition from the hospital to the home environment. The major role of HBHC is to assist with self-care activities and locating community resources, but it is also a welcome link between the supportive environment of the SCI Center and the occasionally overwhelming unfamiliarity of life back in the community.

Personal relationships and community support networks also can be good sources of assistance and moral support in the period following discharge from the hospital. Personal friends and church and special interest groups often are at a loss as to how to assist a person after traumatic injury. In many cases, all that is needed is a call for help and they will rush to be of assistance. It may be difficult to ask for help initially, but the response can be gratifying and a strong source of moral support as you and your family begin to reestablish a normal life.

SUGGESTED READINGS

An Introduction to Spinal Cord Injury. Paralyzed Veterans of America, 801 Eighteenth St., N.W., Washington, DC 20006.

The Disabled Person and Family Dynamics. Reprint Series No. 1. Accent on Living, P.O. Box 700, Bloomington, IL 61701.

Fallon, B. (1978): *So You're Paralyzed*. Spinal Injuries Association, 126 Albert St., London, England NW1 7NF.

Trieschmann, R. B. (1980): *Spinal Cord Injuries: The Psychological, Social and Vocational Adjustment*. Pergamon Press, Maxwell House, Fairview Park, Elmsford, NY 10523.

CHAPTER 2

What Is a Spinal Cord Injury?

Juan Fonseca, Mark N. Ozer,
Peter Axelson, and Lynn Phillips

Although spinal cord injury is a catastrophic event that thrusts you into the unfamiliar and bewildering world of hospitals, medical technology, and rehabilitation, the final outcome depends on a variety of factors. The skills of your medical and rehabilitation teams and the support of your family and friends are important components, but most important is your willingness to deal effectively with the inevitable changes in your physical condition and lifestyle. In this chapter we will provide you with information about what has happened to you as well as what you can expect from the strange new world of doctors, nurses, therapists, and technicians.

EMERGENCY CARE

While patients and families attempt to make some sense out of an unacceptable and unfamiliar situation, the medical staff are working to minimize the amount of damage. When a spinal cord injury occurs, the immediate goal of the treatment team is to combat shock, to stabilize the patient medically, and to determine the extent of the injuries. Often a spinal cord injury is accompanied by other injuries: internal injuries, broken bones, skin lacerations, or concussions. Consequently, a battery of tests will be performed in the emergency room to de-

7

termine or confirm the extent and urgency of associated injuries. These tests may include:

- *Assessment of vital signs.* Pulse, blood pressure, respiration.
- *Neurological examinations.* State of consciousness and assessment of brain and spinal cord function.
- *Radiological examinations.* X-rays to detect broken bones and any damage to vital organs.
- *Other diagnostic tests.* Depending upon the particular injury, other diagnostic tests may be indicated.

The medical staff also will attempt to identify any preexisting conditions which could complicate the management of the spinal cord injury itself.

The first few hours after injury are the most critical ones from the standpoint of stabilizing your condition and preserving as much function as possible. The most critical factor is to ensure that airways are clear so that breathing can be maintained. The emergency medical team will restore normal breathing as quickly as possible, and other vital signs will be monitored constantly. If blood pressure is low, normal pressure must be reestablished to ensure that the injured spinal cord receives an adequate blood supply—an essential first step toward ensuring that you recover as much function as possible. The longer the blood supply to the cord is reduced, the greater the possibility that function will be impaired.

THE BODY'S REACTION TO INJURY

The traumatic nature of a spinal cord injury causes the body to go into a state called *spinal shock*. In effect, the body simply "shuts down" its normal activities below the level of the injury. Spinal shock occurs immediately after the injury and usually begins to abate in a few days or weeks. Although we don't fully understand what happens when the body is in spinal shock, we do know that the muscles below the level of injury are paralyzed and totally devoid of muscle tone or reflex activity for a period of time.

For example, the bladder must be catheterized because you will not be able to void or you will void involuntarily. Often a Foley indwelling catheter is inserted into the bladder for 2 to 3 days, after which your physician usually will begin a program called *intermittent catheterization.* Intermittent catheterization, or *IC*, consists of catheterizing the patient every 4 to 6 hr so that the bladder can be drained periodically rather than relying on an indwelling catheter. Intermittent catheterization is a time-consuming procedure, but it helps to reduce the danger of bladder infection and can be used to retrain your bladder so that it contracts spontaneously and thus empties itself. Bladder function after SCI is discussed more fully in Chapter 8.

Spinal shock also affects bowel function. In this condition, called *paralytic ileus*, intestinal activity is slowed so that your abdomen may appear distended for the first 3 or 4 days after injury. Once spinal shock begins to subside you will begin to pass gas and feces involuntarily. Once that occurs your treatment team will assist you in developing a regular bowel care program that meets your personal needs. Bowel function is discussed in Chapter 9.

MINIMIZING THE DAMAGE

Once the extent of nerve and bone injury is established, the medical team will try to reduce pressure on the spinal cord so that proper healing can begin. Drugs may be used to reduce the swelling that accompanies and often aggravates the trauma to the spinal cord. Broken spinal vertebrae are treated with traction or immobilization if possible, and surgery may be necessary to decompress the spinal cord at the site of the injury.

Immobilization to promote healing can be accomplished in several ways. If you have a cervical injury, you may be fitted with an immobilizing apparatus called a *halo frame*. The halo (around the head) is attached to a chest and shoulder frame to immobilize the head on the trunk. This device allows you to be mobile in a sitting or standing position early in therapy. Before development of the halo frame, patients were maintained in a horizontal position in traction for 6 to 8 weeks. Although the halo frame usually remains in place for 3 to 4 months, it does not restrict general mobility.

Most newly injured SCI patients are placed on specialized beds that rotate or flip end over end, rather than on standard hospital beds. This allows you to be turned while in traction and protects the skin from pressure sores caused by unremitting pressure on skin over bony prominences.

In short, the goal of the medical team during the immediate period after you have sustained your spinal cord injury is to stabilize your medical condition so that you can achieve maximum return of function. It is helpful, therefore, to know how the spinal cord works so that you can understand not only the problems caused by injury but also the options for active function.

HOW THE SYSTEM WORKS

The spinal cord is part of a very important system of the body called the *nervous system*. The nervous system contributes to every bodily function in some way or another because it is responsible for sending and interpreting the body's messages. You hear, see, feel, and smell not only because your ears, eyes, skin, and nose are responding to sensations, but also because the body somehow is processing those responses. The nervous system, through a very complex process of receiving, interpreting, and sending back messages, coordinates that function.

The nervous system consists of two major parts, the *central nervous system* and the *peripheral nervous system*. The central nervous system is comprised of the brain, optic nerves (eyes), and spinal cord; all other nerves in the body are part of the peripheral nervous system. Peripheral nerves originate primarily in the spinal cord and conduct electrical impulses to and from the rest of the body. The spinal cord then transmits messages to and from the brain.

The brain serves as the thought-processing center for our bodies, but it also processes other kinds of messages. When you cut your finger, for example, the pain that you feel occurs because signals were transmitted from your finger through nerves to the spinal cord and up to the brain, where the brain interpreted those signals as pain. After interpreting the pain signal, the brain sent a signal back down your spinal cord through the peripheral nerves to your finger, where (finally) the sensation of pain was fully realized. While this seems to be a lengthy and complex process, it actually occurs so quickly that we perceive it as one event, even though many complex, interrelated processes are involved.

Sensation, or things that you feel, are carried by *sensory nerves*. Movement, deciding to walk, raise your hand, or move your lips to eat, for example, are controlled by *motor nerves*.

The peripheral nervous system also has nerves that control involuntary body functions such as blood pressure, heartbeat, digestion, body temperature, sweating, and involuntary aspects of urination and sexual function. Such nerves are part of the *autonomic nervous system.*

WHAT HAPPENS AFTER INJURY

The processes involved in transmitting messages throughout the body are fundamentally disrupted when the spinal cord becomes injured. Suddenly, messages from areas below the level of injury no longer can get to the brain nor can the brain send messages to the body below that level. Consequently, all kinds of nerve input—sensory, motor, and autonomic function—to and from the area below the spinal cord lesion are affected.

Injuries to most parts of the body are repairable. If you

break your leg, for example, the cells in the broken bone will begin to repair the area of the break so that you will be able to use that leg. A cut in your finger will heal because your body makes new skin cells to heal the area of the injury. Even the nerves in your finger, which are peripheral nerves, often heal if they become damaged. For reasons that no one really understands, the central nervous system does *not* repair itself when damaged (see Chapter 17 for more information on research to find a cure for spinal cord injury), which is why a spinal cord injury or any other injury to the central nervous system is very serious.

DETERMINING THE EXTENT OF DAMAGE

One of the most important steps after injury is to determine the severity of the injury. Since a spinal cord injury affects sensory, motor, and autonomic function below the level of the injury, its exact location has important implications and determines how much function has been lost. In general, the higher the level of the lesion, the greater the loss of function. Conversely, injuries to lower levels of the spinal cord will affect fewer bodily functions (see Chapter 3 for a full discussion of functional deficit at each level).

Figures 2.1 and 2.2 shows how spinal cord injuries are classified. A spinal cord injury is given a letter and number designation that corresponds to the level of the spinal cord below which nerve injury, or *neurological deficit*, has occurred. As the figure shows, there are four major areas of the spinal cord: cervical, thoracic, lumbar, and sacral.

When the spinal cord is injured at the thoracic or lumbar level, the injury is described as *paraplegia*, because sensation and motor function in the lower part of the body and both legs will be affected. If part or all sensation in arms and fingers is lost, the injury is called *quadriplegia* and all four extremities usually are affected to some extent.

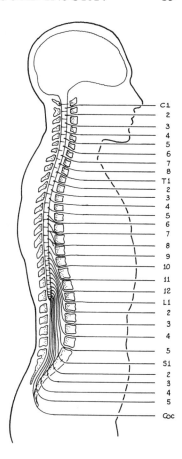

C1
2
3
4
5
6
7
8
T1
2
3
4
5
6
7
8
9
10
11
12
L1
2
3
4
5
S1
2
3
4
5
Coc

FIG. 2.1. Levels at which spinal cord injury can occur.

EFFECTS OF SCI

The two factors that most influence the outcome of spinal cord injury are the *level* at which the injury occurs and the *completeness* of the injury. The level of injury is important because, in general, the higher the lesion, the greater the loss of function. Urinary, bowel, and sexual function will be impaired to some extent in every spinal cord injury because these functions are controlled at the lower levels of the spinal cord. The small muscles that control fine hand function receive their

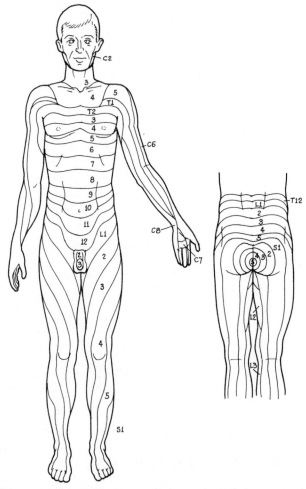

FIG. 2.2. The loss of sensation that occurs below a given level of injury (see Fig. 2.1) is illustrated.

messages from nerves located in the region between C8 and T1, so injuries to that area will have some effect on hand function. Other arm muscles that may be affected include the *extensor* muscles of the forearm (C7) that help to extend your arm, the *flexors* (C6) that help to bring your arm in to the body, and the big shoulder muscles that control the upper arm (C5).

Breathing depends on two sets of muscles: those between the ribs (*intercostals*); the accessory muscles such as some in the neck, shoulder, and chest; and most importantly the *diaphragm* which provides 60 percent of the exertion necessary for breathing. The intercostal muscles that expand and contract the chest cavity are supplied by T1 to T12, so their usefulness is lost in cervical and high thoracic lesions. The accessory muscles are supplied with nerve impulses from high in the thoracic and cervical regions of the cord.

The diaphragm, which separates the chest from the abdomen, has an unusual nerve supply, the *phrenic nerve*, which originates from C2 to C4. Fortunately, because it depends on nerves so high in the system, diaphragm breathing is preserved in all but the highest lesions.

If the diaphragm itself is affected by an injury at the higher cervical levels, a respirator can be used to support breathing function. In some cases, people with injuries that affect breathing can have *phrenic nerve stimulators* implanted to allow them to breath all or part of the time without the aid of a respirator. A physician will be able to tell you whether phrenic nerve stimulation is appropriate for your particular injury.

If your injury occurred above the level of T8, your body's ability to regulate temperature and blood pressure can be seriously affected. This can lead to a complication called *autonomic dysreflexia*, in which your blood pressure may rise to very high levels. If not treated, autonomic dysreflexia can be life-threatening, so it is important to understand its causes and treat it immediately if it does occur (see Chapter 11).

The completeness of a spinal cord injury helps to determine how much function will be maintained. When injury is complete there is no measurable neurologic function at and below the level of the cord damage, and usually no movement or sensation below the level of injury. When injury is incomplete (and approximately one-half of all spinal cord injuries are incomplete), some sensation or movement is retained below the level of injury. This can range from the ability to perceive touch in certain areas to almost complete functional recovery. Incomplete paralysis occurs most often in lesions in the cervical area, whereas most complete lesions occur at the lower levels. Therefore, the probability of improvement of function is more likely in cervical injuries. Total lack of response to a pinprick or touch in the area of the scrotum, penis, or anus or no conscious control of the anal sphincter are indications that the lesion probably is complete. Conversely, any sensation or conscious motor control indicates that the lesion probably is incomplete.

HOW NERVES WORK

The nerves that supply each level of the spinal cord occur in pairs. One nerve conducts messages from the body to the brain, while the paired nerve carries the messages from the brain to the body. In all, there are 31 of these "nerve pairs," with one pair for each neurological level. The nerve that carries messages from the body to the brain carries *sensory* impulses. The brain reacts to those impulses with a *motor* response. If, for example, you place your leg against a hot pipe, the sensory nerve endings at that location say, "Too hot!" That message is conducted via the spinal cord to your brain, which responds by sending a message back that says "Move your legs away from that pipe." All this information is transmitted so fast that it may seem to be one message, but in fact there is sensory input (one message) and a motor response (a second message).

When the spinal cord—the courier for those messages—is disrupted at or above the level of T12 this paired message system also is interrupted. Your brain may tell your leg to move, but that message gets only as far as the spinal cord injury. Likewise, your leg may be trying to tell your brain, "Too hot!" so that it will send back a motor message telling your leg to move, but the sensory message stops at the site of the injury. Since the nerves supplying the body have no way to "understand" what is going on when their only message system is interrupted, the messages shoot back and forth below the level of the lesion, creating a loop of nerve impulses that result in *spasticity*, which is described in greater detail in Chapter 11. A positive effect of spasticity is that it helps to maintain muscle tone and increased blood circulation. Sometimes spasticity can be directed to assist with functional activities such as standing.

Injuries that occur below the level of T12 are described more accurately as injuries to the *cauda equina* rather than as spinal cord injuries. In these lesions, the injury interrupts *all* reflex activity, which means that no messages can be carried back and forth as with higher levels of injury. Since all reflex action is interrupted, the paralysis is called *flaccid paralysis*, because the body has no way to maintain muscle tone or muscle activity.

In the upcoming chapters, we will look at the physical effects of spinal cord injury, and examine the kinds of function that are possible after injury and the methods that you can use to achieve these functions. We also will look at other aspects of life after injury that may be worrying you. Although a spinal cord injury may at first appear to be overwhelming, it is likely that you will be able to regain much more independence than you currently believe is possible. Armed with knowledge about how your body works, a desire to obtain as much function as possible for a given level of injury, and ideas for dealing with what may appear to be insurmountable barriers, you can discover ways to participate in a wide range of activities that will help you feel good again about life.

SUGGESTED READINGS

Donovan, W. H., and Bedbrook, Sir G. (1982): Comprehensive management of spinal cord injury. *Clinical Symposia,* 34(2). CIBA Pharmaceutical Company, CIBA-GEIGY Corp., Summit, NJ 07901.

Ireland, F.: *Spinal Cord Injury Care Manual for Nurses.* Eastern Paralyzed Veterans Association, 432 Park Ave. South, New York, NY 10016.

Krenzel, J. R., and Rohrer, L. M. (1977): *Paraplegic and Quadriplegic Individuals—Handbook of Care for Nurses.* National Spinal Cord Injury Association, 149 California St., Newton, MA 02158.

Spinal Cord Injury Handbook. Craig Hospital, 3425 South Clarkson, Englewood, CO 80110.

CHAPTER 3

Rehabilitation

Lynn Phillips

The purpose of rehabilitation is to enable a person to resume an active and satisfying life after spinal cord injury. When a person first enters the acute care hospital, the goal of the medical team is to minimize the amount of impairment that will result from the injury. The goal of rehabilitation is to minimize the amount of disability that will occur as a result of physical impairment. Consequently, a rehabilitation program focuses on physical retraining and strengthening, bladder and bowel management, mobility, psychosocial aspects of reacting to injury, and the transition from a hospital environment to home. Although rehabilitation can and will continue after you leave the hospital, this chapter focuses on the rehabilitation that takes place in a hospital or rehabilitation center.

CHOOSING A REHABILITATION PROGRAM

One of the most important decisions you will make shortly after injury is where you will receive your rehabilitation. Although you had little or no choice about where you were hospitalized immediately after your accident, the rehabilitation phase usually is a more positive experience if you are able to go to a center that specializes in rehabilitation. Consequently, you will want to participate fully in deciding where you will go. To do so, you will need a working knowledge of the different kinds of rehabilitation programs available. Armed with this knowledge, the program you enter is most likely to be able to address your particular needs.

WHERE TO LOOK

The federal Rehabilitation Services Administration (RSA) established a series of Model Regional SCI Treatment Centers throughout the United States in the early 1970s to encourage excellence in the care and treatment of spinal cord–injured patients. These centers are located in the "hubs" of certain geographic regions and receive federal funding for research and training in the area of spinal cord injury. As of 1986 there were 13 such centers.

Veterans may be eligible for free medical care and rehabilitation through 1 of the 20 Veterans Administration's Spinal Cord Injury Centers. The VA was the first agency in this country to develop specialized centers for spinal cord injury care, where military veterans who can demonstrate financial need are treated without charge. Veterans who are in need of spinal cord rehabilitation services should contact one of the VA SCI Centers (Appendix 1) or a Paralyzed Veterans of America service officer (Appendix 2) as soon as possible after injury to determine their eligibility for VA medical care. Other excellent rehabilitation and SCI treatment centers exist outside of the RSA and VA SCI centers.

FACTORS TO CONSIDER

The period immediately after a catastrophic injury can be confusing and mentally exhausting. At times of extreme stress many of us have a tendency to avoid making decisions rather than to take advantage of the alternatives that are available. Choosing a rehabilitation facility is one of the choices that many newly injured people and their families leave to the attending physician or admitting hospital. Although their advice can be helpful, it is beneficial to both patient and family to examine some of the alternatives available and to weigh the factors that influence the choice of facility.

A major consideration is the *quality of medical care* available at a given facility, and the opinions of the attending physician are helpful in evaluating this aspect. The opinions of other physicians and consultation with a local independent living center will further assist in ensuring that the best possible medical care is obtained.

A second consideration is the *attitude and philosophy* toward rehabilitation at any given facility. Surprisingly, this can vary dramatically; some rehabilitation centers pursue maximum functional recovery much more aggressively than do others, and the personnel take a more optimistic approach. Some use a traditional medical model of treatment, whereas others stress group living and encourage informal interaction among patients and staff. Attitude and philosophy are difficult qualities to quantify, but they can be extremely important factors in evaluating the effectiveness of a rehabilitation program. Here again, local organizations of citizens with disabilities can be a valuable source of information; they have been through the system and can provide practical advice based on firsthand experiences.

A third major factor is *cost*. With the exception of the VA Spinal Cord Injury Centers, all rehabilitation programs mentioned in this book charge for their services. Although most rehabilitation programs will be covered to some extent by standard health insurance policies, most insurance coverage is limited to a maximum number of days; thus, an estimate of the length of inpatient rehabilitation that will be needed will be helpful. You will want to know what happens when insurance coverage ceases. Will the rehabilitation program be completed by that time, and, if not, who is responsible for paying the balance?

Another important consideration is *geographic location*. The family can be an important component of the rehabilitation team if they are able to participate actively. By being involved in the rehabilitation process on a day-to-day basis, family members become knowledgeable about the physical and psychological aspects of recovery from a devastating injury. Again, this factor must be weighed against the others—medical care, philosophy and attitude, and cost—in determining which rehabilitation center is "best" for a particular individual.

A critical factor in choosing a rehabilitation program is the staff's knowledge and experience with spinal cord injury. Medical personnel in community hospitals who see only five or six SCI patients per year rarely have the expertise necessary to assist spinal cord–injured individuals maximize their potential. Even some large metropolitan hospitals cannot offer the full range of services to be found in specialized treatment centers. Therefore, if your physician or hospital administrator does not mention the availability of comprehensive rehabilitation centers to you, you should explore them yourself. It is important to realize that it may be difficult for physicians and administrators to admit that other facilities can provide better care than they can, especially in these days of economic competition for patients. In the collective opinion of many people with spinal cord injuries and professionals in this field, appropriate care can best be provided at a facility that specializes in spinal cord injury rehabilitation. It is important to seek information from those currently living with a spinal injury in the community to supplement the information you receive from professionals. You may wish to call some of the facilities listed in Appendix 1 for specific information about their programs.

PHYSICAL POTENTIAL

Almost all human beings, with and without disabilities, operate at a level that is considerably less than their maximum physical potential. A grossly overweight, sedentary male of

65 who smokes three packs of cigarettes a day and drinks himself to sleep each night clearly is not taking advantage of his maximum physical potential; a body builder such as Arnold Schwarzenegger probably operates close to his maximum physical potential. Thus, there is a continuum, and most of us fall somewhere in between these two extremes.

The continuum exists because the people involved make conscious personal choices about what they expect of themselves physically. Whether one is "able-bodied" (a category that includes both the overweight male of 65 and Arnold Schwarzenegger) or "disabled" (a category that includes wheelchair athletes as well as sedentary disabled persons), individuals have any number of choices about how physically fit they would like to be, given whatever physical capabilities exist.

Because of the wide variation in personal expectations for physical ability, and because no two spinal cord injuries are the same, it is extremely difficult to predict with any degree of accuracy how much function a given individual will recover. The severity of the injury, including the level of lesion and whether the lesion was complete or incomplete, clearly is one significant factor in determining how much function and sensation a person will recover. Equally important, though, is the physical and mental commitment that the individual makes to maximizing whatever function remains.

Although recovery of function is not predictable, some general guidelines have been developed that give an indication of the level of functional recovery that can reasonably be expected with a given level of injury. According to William H. Donovan, M.D.,[1] recovery of function generally follows the pattern listed below for each level of injury indicated.

---

[1] W. H. Donovan, (1981): In *Handbook of Severe Disability*, edited by W. C. Stolov and M. R. Clowers, pp. 70, 71. U.S. Department of Education, Rehabilitation Services Administration, Washington, D.C.

Sacral (S2, S3, S4) Levels

Only bowel and bladder functions are initially impaired with injuries at these levels, and with appropriate treatment you can obtain complete independence in the execution of these functions.

Lumbosacral (L5, S1, S2) Levels

Initially, bowel, bladder, and walking functions are impaired. Complete independence in bowel and bladder function is achieved through appropriate treatment. Independence in walking is also restored with the assistance of two canes or two crutches and sometimes short leg braces (ankle-foot orthoses). Prolonged standing may remain impaired. No wheelchair is necessary.

Lumbar (L1, L2, L3, L4) Levels

Initially, bowel, bladder, and ambulation functions are impaired. With treatment, bowel and bladder function can become independent. Walking can become independent for short distances. Wheelchairs are also used, and complete independence is possible.

Thoracic (T7–T12) Levels

Initially, personal hygiene, ambulation, transfers, dressing, and driving are impaired. Complete independence in bowel and bladder function can be achieved. Independent walking is usually used only for exercise, and complete independence in wheelchair ambulation is accomplished. With training, transfers, dressing, and driving become independent.

Thoracic (T2–T6) Levels

Initially, personal hygiene, ambulation, transfers, dressing, and driving are impaired. With rehabilitation, independence in all these functions is possible. Ambulation is accomplished by use of a wheelchair.

Cervical (C7, C8, T1) Levels

Initially, personal hygiene, ambulation, transfers, eating, dressing, writing, and driving are impaired. Almost all people with injuries at this level become completely independent in all functions consistent with living alone. Independent ambulation is by wheelchair. For some people, however, personal hygiene may require partial physical assistance, transfers may require standby assistance; and dressing may require partial physical assistance.

Cervical (C6) Level

Initially, all functions are impaired. Only a small number of people with injuries at this level are able to achieve complete independence in all functions, and the majority require partial physical assistance for personal hygiene. Wheelchair ambulation is independent. Transfers may require standby assistance and dressing usually requires partial physical assistance. Complete independence is achieved in eating, writing (although slower than usual), and driving.

Cervical (C5) Level

Initially, all functions are impaired. With extensive rehabilitation independence in powered wheelchair ambulation is achieved and nearly full eating skills are achieved. Physical dependence remains for personal hygiene, transfers, dressing, writing, and driving.

Cervical (above C5) Level

Initially, all functions are impaired. In addition, breathing is severely compromised. Training in the use of special respiratory equipment usually is required. The individual is physically dependent for most functions, although some self-propulsion in a powered wheelchair is possible. Devices such as environmental control units, robotic arms, and other electronic aids also can increase independence.

In addition, genital sexual function is impaired to some extent at all levels (see Chapter 12 for an in-depth discussion of this topic).

PHYSICAL THERAPY

One of the most important keys to maximizing physical potential is your physical therapy (PT) program. The physical therapist will assess your physical abilities and will develop an exercise program that will help you achieve your highest possible level of physical potential. A good therapy program also will help to prevent complications that can occur as a result of a spinal injury.

During the first few days after an injury, a physical therapist generally performs *range of motion* (ROM) exercises on the individual. These are passive exercises in which the therapist manually moves your arms and legs in repetitive movements to stimulate circulation, maintain flexibility of the joints, and keep the muscles in relatively good condition. Without ROM exercises, side effects such as poor circulation, blood clots, or pressure sores can occur. Lack of movement also can cause muscles to atrophy or lose their muscle tone and can cause joints to become immobile. Consequently, regular scheduled ROM sessions are vital to maintaining the body's functions during the earliest stages after injury and for the rest of your life. In some cases, family members will be trained in ROM exercises so that the passive exercise program can continue after you return home. In most cases, you will perform ROM yourself.

As soon as it is physically possible, you will be expected to participate actively in a physical reconditioning program. Physical therapy provides you with the skills and equipment necessary for optimum return of function, as well as alternative ways of accomplishing those activities that cannot be done as they once were.

Throughout a physical rehabilitation program, physicians, nurses, and therapists continue to assess and reassess functional capabilities. Some people, after recovering from the initial spinal shock, exhibit greater return of function than originally expected. Others, through sheer effort of will and persistence, also progress more quickly than anticipated. Still others, troubled by problems related to the injury, may progress less quickly than initially had been expected. However, you can participate actively in this continuing assessment of function by keeping track of sensation and movement that returns and by working with the professional treatment team to use this return of function in exercise programs and in daily activities. Thus you must realize that each person is unique and it may be unnecessarily distressing to assess your progress against that of others in the program.

OCCUPATIONAL THERAPY

A discipline closely related to physical therapy yet unique unto itself is occupational therapy (OT). The occupational therapist helps to bridge the gap between the function that has been reattained through physical therapy and the function that is needed to carry on the activities of daily living (ADL). Sometimes this is achieved by teaching new ways of accomplishing old tasks; at other times it is achieved by using adaptive devices or equipment. Occupational therapists can assist you in determining what can be done without assistance, which activities will require assistance, and what kinds of devices will enable you to perform specific functions. It is very important that you specifically describe the types of activities that you would like to accomplish so that your OT can help you achieve your goals to the extent possible.

NURSING AND SCI

A nurse often is the single most important staff member to a person with a spinal cord injury because the nursing staff is there when you are the most helpless and providing the specialized care that is so important. In addition, the nursing staff assists SCI patients in putting to use the skills and techniques that have been learned in physical and occupational therapy, such as transferring from bed to wheelchair, getting dressed, and learning how to bathe and groom yourself after a spinal cord injury. Bowel and bladder training programs also are learned and practiced with the assistance of the nursing staff.

Because of the close daily contact between SCI patients and their nurses, nurses often are asked the questions that arise as a result of attempting new activities after injury. With their specialized training, nurses in spinal cord injury and rehabilitation centers are excellent resources for every aspect of SCI. And, if they don't know the answers, they usually know where to find them.

In many facilities, the nursing staff manages, or at least participates actively in, a patient education program. The purpose of patient education is to provide newly injured persons with information about spinal cord injury, as well as to provide an opportunity to discuss areas of concern with other patients and with staff members. Most SCI centers have developed special education materials for their patient education classes, including films, videotapes, and home care manuals.

ACTIVITIES OF DAILY LIVING

Learning how to perform the activities of daily living after injury is one of the most important steps in a personal rehabilitation process. Activities of daily living skills include:

1. Bladder care
2. Bowel care

3. Prevention of pressure sores
4. Bathing
5. Dressing
6. Grooming
7. Transferring from bed to wheelchair and back
8. Eating
9. Cooking
10. Housecleaning

Activities of daily living can be performed independently, with mechanical assistance, or with personal assistance from attendants or family members. How much can be done without assistance from others is determined both by the level of injury and by personal ingenuity in modifying those activities. For an indication of what activities generally can be performed for each level of injury, refer to the list beginning on page 24.

BLADDER CARE

Bladder and kidney problems can be one of the most serious side effects of spinal cord injury. However, early establishment of an acceptable bladder management program can minimize the health risks to a person with paraplegia or quadriplegia. In addition, establishment of a regularly scheduled program leads to increased independence, because scheduled elimination makes it easier to participate in regular daily activities, such as recreation, employment, and socializing.

Immediately after injury, the attending physician probably will recommend that urinary drainage be accomplished with the use of an indwelling Foley catheter. However, many facilities now begin as soon after injury as possible to use a system of bladder management called *intermittent catheterization*, in which a catheter is inserted into the bladder at regularly scheduled intervals. Bladder management is discussed fully in Chapter 8.

BOWEL CARE

The bowels are affected by injury in much the same manner as the bladder. Immediately after the injury, spinal shock prevents the bowels from moving spontaneously. Thus bowel movements need to be stimulated either with suppositories, laxatives, digital stimulation, or a combination of these methods.

As spinal shock begins to resolve, many find that the act of getting onto a toilet provides the physical and psychological stimulation necessary to activate the elimination process. For others, digital stimulation, laxatives, or suppositories may be necessary. Again, the kind as well as the degree of stimulation will be determined by the level of lesion and by the individual. Bowel management is discussed fully in Chapter 9.

SUMMARY

Inpatient rehabilitation will provide multiple opportunities to discuss with staff and other patients the feelings that go along with onset of a new injury and to explore questions about life after injury. How do I get into my house? Will I be able to work again? How will other people respond to me now that I am in a wheelchair? These kinds of questions are addressed in greater detail in later chapters.

A good, comprehensive rehabilitation program can do much to provide a newly injured person with the information and skills necessary to make living with a disability easier. It also can be a period in which to develop physical capabilities to the highest extent possible. The success of any rehabilitation program, though, is very much dependent on your own efforts and your willingness to continue the process after returning home. A university, for example, can provide exciting courses, good professors, and excellent resources for the inquiring student. For a student to get the maximum benefit out of that university, however, she or he must be committed to studying and taking advantage of the resources provided.

An analogous situation occurs during a rehabilitation process. You can participate fully and take advantage of available resources or you can remain fairly passive and let "them"— the professional staff—attempt rehabilitation. It is fairly obvious that the most benefit will occur if you participate actively and aggressively in the process.

Personal motivation can be difficult when the anticipated outcome is something short of complete recovery of function. The alternative, though, is even less recovery of function and over a longer period of time.

Rehabilitation is not an easy process. It requires concentrated physical effort, determination, and the need to confront many fears and anxieties. It is, however, an essential segment of the process leading to reentry to the world at large and reestablishing your own goals, hopes, and desires for the future.

SUGGESTED READINGS

Burke, D. C., and Murray, D. D. (1975): *Handbook of Spinal Cord Medicine,* Raven Press, New York.

Power, P. W., and Dell Orto, A. E. (eds.): *The Role of the Family in the Rehabilitation of the Physically Disabled.* Pro-Ed Publishers, 5341 Industrial Oaks Blvd., Austin, TX 78735.

The Realities of Spinal Cord Injury. Sacred Heart Rehabilitation Hospital, 1545 S. Layton Blvd., Milwaukee, WI 53215.

Rossier, A. B. (reprint 1975): *Rehabilitation of the Spinal Cord Injury Patient.* Pharmaceuticals Division, CIBA-GEIGY Corp., Summit, NJ.

Wright, G. N. (1980): *Total Rehabilitation.* Little, Brown and Co., Boston, MA.

CHAPTER 4

Mobility

Lynn Phillips

A practical problem resulting from spinal cord injury is mobility, that is, simply "getting around." Before your injury, you used a variety of techniques to get from one place to another. You would walk, drive a car, take a train, ride in a boat, or fly by plane. Some people use a tractor to plow a field or skis to get down a hill or a chair with wheels to grab something a few feet from a desk. Everyday we all accomplish mobility in a variety of ways. The means used to achieve mobility depend on where we are going, how far it is, and how fast we want to get there. In many cases, the way you will get from one place to another for longer distances will be essentially the same as the way you got there before the injury, i.e., by car or plane. The major mobility difference now is the method you will use to go shorter distances, those places to which you used to walk.

TO WALK OR USE A WHEELCHAIR

A question that many people with new spinal cord injuries ask is, "Will I walk again?" The answer depends on the severity of the injury, the amount of energy needed to walk with braces and/or crutches or a cane, and your own personal feelings about the costs and benefits of walking versus using a wheelchair.

Technically, most paraplegics with a lesion below the level

of T7 can walk with the use of braces and crutches. Some quadriplegics, such as those with fairly incomplete lesions also are able to walk to some extent. Whether one chooses to walk as a regular means of mobility depends on the factors outlined above.

For example, a highly successful businessman with quadriplegia runs a major national enterprise, supervises almost 100 employees in offices throughout the country, and often travels to meetings in other states. He *can* walk but has chosen to use a wheelchair for mobility because his lifestyle is too active for him to be slowed down by the effort required to walk. Another person with paraplegia uses braces and crutches exclusively; although the energy expended to walk with braces and crutches is significantly greater than it would be if he used a wheelchair, he feels that walking is worth the extra effort.

Each of these individuals has evaluated his own mobility requirements and preferences and chosen the "right" method for his lifestyle and needs. These decisions are highly personal, and may change over time as your needs and circumstances change. Furthermore, there are many points within the walk/don't walk continuum. You may choose to use a wheelchair some of the time and walk at other times. If you have quadriplegia your energy expenditure choice may be between a manual or a powered wheelchair. Again, what you decide will depend on your lifestyle, your feelings, and your cost: benefit analysis of energy expenditure and other factors.

You are the only qualified decision maker. Walking with braces and crutches is not intrinsically better than using a wheelchair, nor is using a wheelchair necessarily better than using braces and crutches. Both are a means to an end; getting to where you want to go in a manner most acceptable to you.

WHEELCHAIR MOBILITY

Most people who have a spinal cord injury use a wheelchair (Fig. 4.1) for mobility, either because of physical inability to

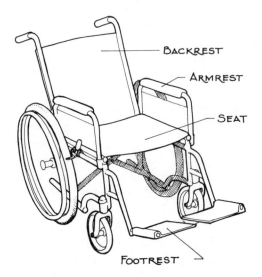

FIG. 4.1. Standard manual wheelchair.

walk effectively with assistive devices or because the energy costs exceed the benefits. Inasmuch as wheelchair usage probably will be an integral part of your life, it is important to select a mobility system that requires minimum energy expenditure and maximum freedom. Thus, the process of choosing a wheelchair and seating system is an important one in which you must evaluate your needs in conjunction with the kinds of equipment—wheelchairs, seating systems, method of propulsion, and various add-on equipment—that are available.

Before talking with a physician or therapist about the products that are on the market, you should consider the daily routine that you had before your injury and what aspects of that routine may be important to wheelchair selection. Just as we all have different needs and desires in the kinds of cars we drive, so will individuals have different needs in a wheelchair. Is your lifestyle a fairly mobile one, or is it more sedentary than most? Are you going to school, or do you have to travel quite a bit for your job? Do you spend most of your

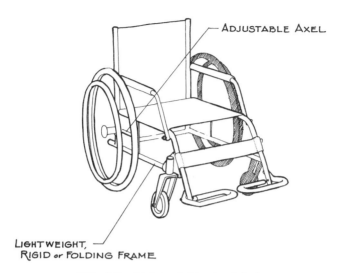

ADJUSTABLE AXEL

LIGHTWEIGHT, RIGID or FOLDING FRAME

FIG. 4.2. Lightweight wheelchair.

days behind a desk? How you spend your time will give you some idea of the features you will need in a wheelchair. If you move around a lot during the day, such as traveling across a college campus to classes, a lightweight wheelchair (Fig. 4.2) may be high on your list of priorities, because a lightweight chair reduces the amount of energy required to get around. If you anticipate getting into and out of a car fairly often, another important feature will be how easy it is to take the chair with you.

In addition to considering your personal preferences and lifestyle, the severity of your disability is an important consideration in selecting a wheelchair. Wheelchairs commonly used by people with spinal cord injuries include the newer, sporty, low-back chairs that are hand-propelled; the more traditional, high-back chairs that also are propelled manually; three-wheeled, powered platforms; and traditional powered wheelchairs (Fig. 4.3) with four wheels, high backs, and a power source located underneath the seat. Although there are

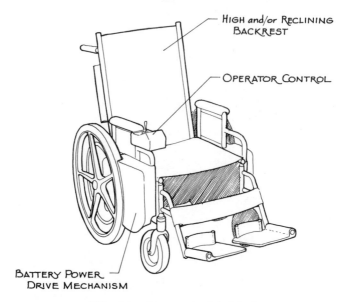

HIGH and/or RECLINING BACKREST

OPERATOR CONTROL

BATTERY POWER DRIVE MECHANISM

FIG. 4.3. Powered wheelchair.

other reasons for your selection of chair, a major consideration should be how much assistance you need from a wheelchair. If you are healthy, in good physical shape, and are disabled at a relatively low spinal level, in all likelihood you would not want a powered wheelchair. If, on the other hand, you are a fairly high-level quadriplegic, you probably will require such a chair.

An excellent source of information about wheelchairs and wheelchair selection is other users. Talk to people who have used a wheelchair for several years and find out what they do and do not like about their chairs. Ask them what features they will look for in a wheelchair when it is time to replace the one they are using now. Someone who uses a wheelchair day in and day out can be an invaluable resource to someone who has never before considered the relative merits of wheelchairs.

It is equally important to make sure that your wheelchair is the appropriate size and configuration to fit your body. Wheelchairs for adults generally have seat widths from 16 to 18 inches, a seat depth (front to back of the chair) of 16 inches, and seats that are situated approximately 20 inches from the floor. However, wider or narrower chairs are available, and other dimensions can vary as well. It is *essential* that your wheelchair fit your body so that additional physical problems such as scoliosis (curvature of the spine), pressure sores, and arthritis can be prevented.

Most wheelchairs have footrests, armrests, and backrests to provide additional support and stability. Proper fit of these accessories is just as important as is proper fit of the seating surface. If footrests are too low, your feet and legs will not receive the proper support to maintain good muscle tone and circulation. Inadequate back support can lead to instability if you have difficulty maintaining your balance. Armrests that are too high obstruct the motion needed to use the handrims on the wheels, and thus interfere with your ability to propel the wheelchair. Some individuals with fairly good balance and low-level lesions prefer chairs with no armrests because armrests increase the weight of the chair, limit how far underneath a table or desk the chair will go, and limit how far you can reach.

ACCESSORIES

Other features to consider are those that provide specialized function. Some wheelchairs have a seat that raises the user into a standing position. Others have power sources which elevate the entire seat (still in sitting position) to a higher level. Some chairs have special attachments which assist the user in climbing curbs or steps. When selecting a chair, careful consideration of all options is important to ensure that your chair meets your needs.

POWERED WHEELCHAIRS

A powered wheelchair often will be required by someone with limited upper body strength. Depending on the degree of disability, the powered chair may be fitted with a variety of accessories to increase independence and mobility. Powered reclining systems can allow you to change position without assistance. A tray table can be placed across your lap to provide a surface for writing and eating and to provide support for the arms and hands. If you rely on a respirator for breathing support, that system can be attached to the chair.

Powered wheelchairs can be controlled by whatever method is most convenient and most acceptable to you. Some people are able to use a joystick mounted near the armrest. Others may require or prefer a "sip and puff" device controlled by the mouth or a chin-controlled joystick. Additional control systems are available for people who need them.

Since many users of powered wheelchairs may require several accessory devices to maximize their levels of independence, the wheelchair and all add-ons should be purchased together so that a well-coordinated mobility system is developed. Whatever your needs are, it is vitally important that you are intimately involved in the discussions, and that you know what alternatives are available and what the costs and benefits will be.

SELECTING YOUR WHEELCHAIR

Once you have determined your preferences regarding the features, style, and level of assistance you want in a wheelchair, it is time to look at the various products available. Within the past 10 years, the variety of wheelchairs and accessory equipment has increased dramatically so that you should be able to order a chair that closely meets your personal needs. In addition to obtaining information about wheelchair availability from your therapist, look through publications like

Paraplegia News, Accent on Living, and *Sports'n Spokes* for articles and advertisements about new wheelchair design. You probably will be surprised by the number of options available to you.

WHEELCHAIR MAINTENANCE

To provide maximum service to the user, wheelchairs require regular maintenance and care, just like any other piece of equipment. If you do not maintain your chair, small problems are likely to become large ones and your wheelchair will tend to wear out quickly. With proper maintenance and proper use, your wheelchair should last for a long time.

Most wheelchair manufacturers provide each purchaser with a booklet that explains how to keep the chair in shape. Become familiar with the parts of your chair and follow the procedures outlined for keeping it in good condition.

Wheelchairs generally are used both indoors and out and, like any other equipment that goes outdoors, they will come into contact with dirt, grease, grime, and salt. Wheelchairs should be kept clean so that this kind of debris does not interfere with nuts, bolts, and bearings. Tires should be kept inflated at an appropriate pressure to allow for ease of movement as well as proper maintenance. All contact points between different parts of the chair—those places where screws, nuts, and bolts hold the chair together—should be checked regularly to make sure that each section is fastened tightly to the next. Wheelchairs are relatively sturdy objects, but a chair's reliability is dependent as much on the user's care and upkeep as it is on the chair itself.

Few people would buy a car without thinking first of features they desire, style that appeals to them, or comfort of the vehicle, yet many people with new injuries take a passive role when it comes to choosing a wheelchair by assuming that the therapist or physician will prescribe what is "best" for them. Therapists and physicians do not know enough about you, your needs, or your interests to make all the decisions. Again, to ensure that your chair will be the best one for you, it pays to be actively involved in the decision process and well informed beforehand about the options available.

WHEELCHAIR CUSHIONS

An essential component of a wheelchair mobility system, whether you use a manual or a powered wheelchair, is the seating system. In many cases, the seating system consists primarily of a cushion placed on the seat to prevent pressure sores and to assist you in other aspects of wheelchair seating, such as mobility and stability. A good cushion can provide important postural support, help place you at the right height in your chair for maximum function with minimum effort, and distribute the weight on the buttocks to alleviate pressure on bony prominences. A poor cushion can exacerbate postural problems, over- or undercompensate for an improper seat height, and actually increase the risk of pressure sores by reinforcing pressure on certain areas of the body.

In addition to conforming to your shape and physical needs, the cushion should be appropriate for the kind of wheelchair that has been selected. Wheelchair cushions can range from simple foam rubber to expensive, custom-built systems that include much more than a seating surface. For some people, an inexpensive foam cushion is perfectly adequate, although foam cushions generally last only 4 to 9 months, depending on usage. Others will require more sophisticated seating systems, depending on the level and type of disability, skin quality, the amount of postural support needed, and personal comfort.

For most people with spinal cord injuries, the seating system will be a cushion that is placed on top of the sling seat of the chair. Seat cushions generally consist of an external covering that is washable and moisture-proof and an internal material that provides support and distributes pressure. Cushions can be made out of polyurethane foam, gel, water, air, or small beads of polystyrene. Some cushions include a combination of materials to maximize the positive properties of the various components.

In addition to being made out of a variety of materials, wheelchair cushions come in a number of different shapes. The most common shape is a flat surface that conforms to the shape of the wheelchair seat and is 3 to 5 inches thick. Other cushions are contoured to fit the shape of the human body, and yet another consists of rows of rubber sacs filled with air. All special designs such as these are intended to redistribute pressure.

Some people may require a more comprehensive seating system that provides back and side support in addition to serving the functions of a seat cushion. Several new products have been introduced in recent years which provide that kind of extensive support, although they generally are more expensive than a seat cushion alone would be.

Although manufacturers understandably tout the advantages of their cushion over others and certain hospitals tend to emphasize specific cushions, in truth there is no "ideal" wheelchair cushion. For some people, gel-filled cushions are better than molded foam cushions; in other cases the opposite is true. Air-fllled cushions work well for many people and not as well for others. Factors such as bone size, weight, skin sensitivity, climate, temperature, humidity, and duration of sitting time all need to be considered when selecting a cushion. By working closely with your rehabilitation personnel you will be able to determine which cushion best serves your needs.

BRACES AND CRUTCHES

Some people with spinal cord injuries are able to walk, either for short periods of time or on a regular basis. Walking is usually assisted by a combination of braces and crutches.

The kinds of braces and crutches used depend on the level of injury and the amount and kind of function that remains.

Depending on the level and severity of injury, one of two basic approaches to walking can be used. The most common style is a "swing-through" gait, in which both legs are propelled forward at the same time by placing the crutches in front of your body and swinging your body forward. Other people are able to move one leg forward at a time. The two most commonly used brace systems are the traditional bilateral (both legs) knee, ankle, and foot orthosis with a pelvic band and hip joint locks, and the newer reciprocating gait orthosis that is lighter in weight than standard braces and supposedly requires less effort. Bracing systems are used either with standard underarm crutches or with Canadian crutches that put the weight of the upper body on the arms rather than under the arms.

SUMMARY

How you decide to get around after injury will be based on many factors, including the extent of injury, personal feelings about walking, and the amount of energy you are willing to expend in the process. Before making such a decision, talk to physicians, nurses, and therapists but the best resource will be other people with spinal cord injuries who have been through the same process. Try to find someone who is using braces and crutches or has used them in the past, and find out what they consider to be the costs and benefits of that method of mobility, and do the same for wheelchairs. If you will require a powered wheelchair, ask current users why they use a joystick or a mouthstick or some other method of operating their chair. Whatever you decide, it is desirable to make that decision based on your own needs, perceptions, and expectations, not on those of staff people or family members. And if you find that your circumstances or preferences change in the future you can always make revisions in your equipment.

SUGGESTED READINGS

Fahland, B.: *Wheelchair Selection: More Than Choosing a Chair with Wheels*. American Rehabilitation Foundation, 1800 Chicago Ave., Minneapolis, MN 55404.

Gibson, B., Marshall, D., Smith, K., and Winn, R. (September 1983): The selection of sports wheelchairs. *Paraplegia News*, 37(9):25–28.

Going Places in Your Own Vehicle. Accent Publications, Gillum Rd. and High Drive, P.O. Box 700, Bloomington, IL 61701.

Jay, P. (revised 1984): *Choosing the Best Wheelchair Cushion*. The Royal Association for Disability and Rehabilitation. RESNA, 1101 Connecticut Ave., N.W., Suite 700, Washington, DC 20036.

Lunt, S.: *A Handbook for the Disabled: Ideas and Inventions for Easier Living*. Charles Scribner's Sons, New York, NY.

Nordstrom, C. (April 1983): *Wheelchair Maintenance and Simple Repair*. Woodrow Wilson Rehabilitation Center, Fishersville, VA 22939.

Wheelchairs and Accessories, an Accent Guide. Accent Special Publications, Cheever Publishing Inc., P.O. Box 700, Bloomington, IL 61701.

Wilson, A. B., Jr. (1986): *Wheelchairs: A Prescription Guide*. Rehabilitation Press, Box 3696, Charlottesville, VA 22903.

CHAPTER 5

Going Home

Lynn Phillips

Many people feel a certain amount of anxiety when the time arrives to leave the hospital and begin living life again at home. This chapter will address some of the practical issues that you may face and areas in which questions and possible problems may arise: home accessibility for wheelchair users; financial considerations; going to work or school; and equipment to enhance personal independence. With proper planning and some thought to these areas before leaving the hospital, many potential problems can be avoided.

MAKING YOUR HOME ACCESSIBLE

Before your injury, you may not have noticed that there were six steps up to your front door, eight to your back door, and a full staircase up to the bedrooms in your home. You also may not have realized that the door to your bathroom was only 24 inches wide, or that kitchen cabinets were intended for use while standing, not while sitting in a wheelchair. These are the typical features of home design that many of us take for granted unless we or someone we know begin to use a wheelchair.

Some houses and apartments have relatively few architectural barriers to wheelchair users; others seem to have one barrier after another to be overcome. Therefore, the first step is to evaluate your own home in a systematic way to determine the scope of problems you may face in making your home accessible. In 1980, the American National Standards Institute (ANSI) published specifications for accessibility of buildings by people with physical disabilities.[1] Although the ANSI specifications are comprehensive and provide guidelines for accessibility of all public and private buildings, some of the recommendations are particularly applicable to the home. To assist you in evaluating your own home, we have developed a home accessibility checklist based on the ANSI specifications (Table 5.1).

It is important to look at the checklist in terms of your own mobility and functional limitations to see how serious a particular problem may be for you personally. One man who became paralyzed over 30 years ago has lived in a split-level home ever since his injury. He has to go up six steps from the main level to the level where the bedrooms and bathrooms are; he has to go down six steps from the main level to reach his workshop. How does he do it? He uses braces and crutches at home, both for physical conditioning and for mobility. For him, the preferred method of making his home accessible was to modify his method of mobility rather than to install elevators or ramps or to move to a more "accessible" house.

Another individual owns a townhouse that has two levels. She also wanted to stay in her home after she became disabled, so she installed a chairlift to take her up and down stairs. She keeps a wheelchair at either end of the stairs so that she can transfer into her chair when she arrives at each level.

Besides these two approaches, structural alterations can be made to the home itself to make it more accessible. Structural alterations can be simple and inexpensive or can become very expensive if you want to make extensive changes. The cost will depend as much on your esthetic needs and desires as on

---

[1] *Specifications for Making Buildings and Facilities Accessible to and Useable by Physically Handicapped People*; ANSI 117.1. American National Standards Institute, New York, 1980, p. 68.

TABLE 5.1 *Home accessibility checklist*[a]

Feature	Yes	No

Getting into your home
1. Paths and walkways should be at least 36 in. wide. Most wheelchairs are 27 to 29 in., so 36 in. will allow room for safe maneuvering.
2. Walkways should be made of stable, firm, and nonslip surfaces.
3. Walkways should be continuous and not interrupted by abrupt level changes or steps. Abrupt level changes and steps can be circumvented by construction of a simple ramp (see next section) or by an elevator or platform lift.
4. The surface should be free of manholes, gratings, or other openings in which wheelchair wheels could become caught.

Ramps
1. Ramps should be a minimum of 36 in. wide.
2. The maximum slope should be 1:12 (i.e., 12 in. of length for each 1 in. rise)
3. The maximum rise should be 30 in. If the rise exceeds 30 in., you should build a level platform or landing part of the way up (Fig. 5.1).
4. All landings should be 60 in. long and at least as wide as the ramp.
5. Ramps should have handrails that are made of nonabrasive material and which extend 12 in. beyond the top and bottom of the ramp.

Hallways and floors
1. Hallways should be at least 36 in. wide (48 in. is preferable). Wherever one must turn around, there should be a 5-ft-diameter circle of space. When turning from a 36 in. wide hallway, a door opening should be 36 in. wide.
2. Floors should be stable, firm, and nonslip.
3. Carpet piles should be $\frac{1}{2}$ in. or less.
4. All rugs and mats should be securely fastened. Throw rugs can get caught in wheels.

Bathrooms
1. Doorways should be at least 32 in. wide.
2. Bathrooms should have adequate space for turning (preferably a 5-ft.-diameter circle) so that the wheelchair user can reach all facilities.

TABLE 5.1   *Home accessibility checklist[a] (contd.)*

Feature	Yes	No

Bathrooms (*contd.*)

3. Toilet seats should be at least 15 in. above the floor.
4. A grab bar 36 in. long should be installed 33 to 36 in. from the floor, either on the rear wall or one of the side walls to provide stability for transfer. (Before having grab bars installed, try using the commode to see where grab bars would be most useful for you.)
5. The toilet paper holder should be within easy reach of the toilet and 19 in. above the floor. (The best way to determine proper placement is to sit on the commode and see where the most comfortable placement is.)
6. Cabinets or other obstacles below the sink should be removed so that a wheelchair can be rolled up to the sink. There should be a 30-in. clearance under the sink.
7. Exposed pipes or sharp surfaces under sinks should be insulated or covered.
8. Faucets should be easy to use with one hand.
9. The medicine cabinet should have at least one shelf mounted 44 in. or less above the floor.
10. The tub should have an in-tub seat or seat at the head of the tub.
11. Controls should be easy to use.
12. Tub should be equipped with a hand-held shower spray with a 60-in. hose.
13. Transfer into the tub should be possible without obstruction of enclosure or door tracks.
14. Shower stalls should have a seat mounted 17 to 19 in. above the floor on the wall opposite the controls.

Kitchen

1. Parallel counters should be separated by at least 40 in. of floor space.
2. Allow a minimum of 30 × 48 in. of floor space in front of each appliance, although 19 in. of this may be under the counter or appliance if the lower cabinet is removed.

TABLE 5.1 *Home accessibility checklist[a]* (contd.)

Feature	Yes	No

Kitchen (*contd.*)
  3. Controls and operating mechanisms should be easy to use with one hand without tight grasping or twisting.
  4. Controls should be 48 in. or less above the floor.
  5. A 30-in. wide opening under an adjustable height counter top should be provided if you wish to wheel beneath the counter (Fig. 5.2).
  6. The sink rim should be 34 in. or less above the floor. It should be $6\frac{1}{2}$ in. deep or less, with the space below it at least 30 in. wide and all exposed pipes insulated or covered. (Fig. 5.3).
  7. The oven should be self-cleaning and adjacent to an accessible counter. Control should be located in the front and placed 48 in. or less above the floor.
  8. At least one shelf in each storage cabinet should be 48 in. or less above the floor.

Living area
  1. The living room, dining room, outside areas (patios, balconies, etc.), garage, and at least one bedroom should be accessible to wheelchairs. The clearance beneath the dining room table should be at least 27 to 30 in.
  2. Telephones should be located within reach of the wheelchair user.
  3. A space of at least 30 × 48 in. should be located next to the bed for ease of transfer.

Laundry area
  1. Room should be accessible.
  2. Equipment should be front-loading, easy to use with one hand without tight grasping or twisting, and controls located 48 in. or less above the floor.

[a] Adapted with permission from N. Ruddy, ANSI A117.1 (1980) Survey/Checklist, *Access Information Bulletin*, 1981.

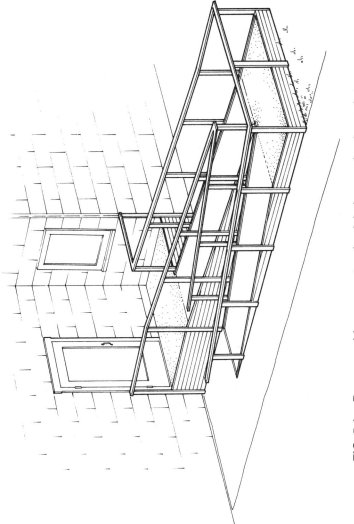

FIG. 5.1. Ramp provides access to wheelchair users in place of steps.

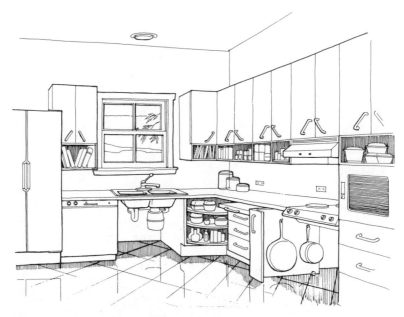

FIG. 5.2. Modifications to kitchens for greater access can increase options for wheelchair users.

the practical needs for access. Information on this rather large subject can be found in the materials cited in the resource list at the end of this chapter.

FINANCIAL CONSIDERATIONS

Money is a major concern for many people after onset of a disability. If the newly disabled family member is the major breadwinner, earnings may be interrupted or cease, depending on the severity of the disability. Medical costs probably will exceed the amount covered by insurance, and lifestyle modifications—making a home accessible, purchasing adaptive equipment, and the possible need for attendant care—can be very expensive.

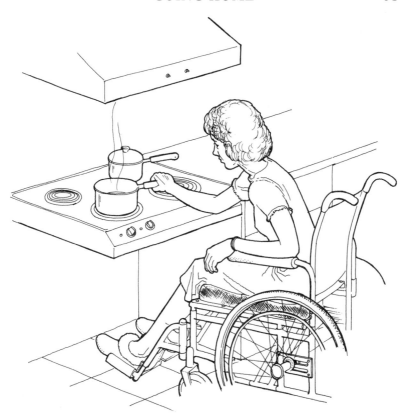

FIG. 5.3. Removing cabinet under stove increases convenience and safety.

A variety of federal, state, and local programs are available to assist people who become spinal cord–injured. Inasmuch as state and local programs vary considerably, it would be wise to check local sources for information about them. Good sources of information about local programs include independent living centers (usually administered by and for disabled persons), rehabilitation centers, the state department of vocational rehabilitation, and consumer-oriented disability groups. Names and addresses of some of these organizations are listed in the appendixes. Organizations and programs not listed can be found in your local telephone book or obtained from state and county social service programs.

Individuals who become injured on the job or in a job-related accident may be eligible for medical care coverage and income support payments through the Workers' Compensation program. This is a federally funded program to which most employers are required to make payments. To find out about benefits to which you may be entitled through Workers' Compensation, contact your state agency.

Active duty military personnel and some ex-military personnel (i.e., those who have served in the armed forces in the past but became disabled after discharge) are eligible for medical care and disability compensation or pension through the Veterans Administration. To find out about VA benefits to which you may be entitled, contact the Veterans Administration regional office closest to you, a Paralyzed Veterans of America Service Office, or any Congressionally chartered veteran's service organization. In addition to providing medical care and income support, the VA conducts job training programs for disabled veterans who want to reenter the work force, as well as other programs of support for which you may qualify. Addresses for VA regional offices and PVA service offices are listed in Appendix II.

The Social Security Administration administers two major income support programs for which severely disabled persons may qualify—Social Security Disability Insurance (SSDI) and Supplemental Security Income (SSI). If you qualify for SSDI benefits, you also will become eligible for Medicare coverage; SSI recipients are eligible for Medicaid coverage.

SSDI eligibility is determined by work history, age, and severity of disability. You must have worked at a job where you contributed to Social Security a minimum number of quarters to qualify for benefits. That minimum number of quarters can range from 6 to 20, depending on the age at which you became disabled. SSDI recipients also must be so severely disabled that, according to the best judgment of the Social Security Administration, they are unable to engage in any substantially gainful activity. Most spinal cord–injured persons who are not working are able to receive SSDI if they have worked enough quarters in covered employment to be eligible. People who receive SSDI also become eligible for Medicare after an initial waiting period. Further information about SSDI and Medicare can be obtained from your local Social Security office.

SSI is a federal income maintenance program for elderly, blind, and disabled persons with financial need. If you have a limited work history or have never worked, do not have any regular means of support, and become disabled as a result of a spinal cord injury, you may qualify for SSI and Medicaid. Again, the local Social Security office is the best place to determine whether you are eligible for these programs.

The other major federal program for disabled persons is the Rehabilitation Services Administration (RSA), the federal agency that oversees each state vocational rehabilitation program. The purpose of vocational rehabilitation is to assist disabled persons enhance their skills so that they will be able to work outside of the home or be a homemaker (see Chapter 3). Vocational rehabilitation can provide job training, job counseling, and, in some instances, adaptive equipment that will enable you to work. Although "voc. rehab." is a federally mandated program, administration and partial funding for the program is the responsibility of each state. Consequently, the best place to find out about a particular state's program is through state government offices.

GOING TO WORK OR SCHOOL

At some time following injury almost everyone faces a variation of the question, "What am I going to do with the rest of my life?" The days and weeks soon after an injury focus on survival and coping with the concept of permanent disability.

Thinking about how you will support yourself and a family can be overwhelming at this point in rehabilitation. If it takes you 20 minutes to get your socks on the first time you try, you may wonder how you can consider a full schedule of classes or working at a job. With each day, however, the basic activities of daily living will take less time, and you will be able to judge more realistically what you can do in a given period of time. By building on these achievements one day at a time, you will begin to see what options are available to you.

Depending on one's age and predisability activities, the future holds many different options. For children, the most obvious option is to return to school, usually the same school attended before the disability occurred. If the classroom is not accessible to wheelchairs, the school has a legal obligation to make it so, either by ensuring that your child's classes are on a floor accessible to wheelchairs or by making modifications to the building itself.

For older children and young adults of college age, returning to school also should not be a problem. Many college campuses have made most or all of their buildings accessible to wheelchairs, and have established special offices to assist disabled students with class scheduling, attendant care, financial aid, and other aspects of college life. Just as important can be the opportunity to share firsthand experiences of college life with others who may have faced similar situations. If you are returning to a college you attended before your injury, contact the disabled students' office before returning so that you can anticipate problems before they occur. If you are in the process of selecting a college, the disabled students' offices can be good resources for determining which school(s) can best accommodate your needs. In short, going to school should be as much an option to you now as it was before you were disabled. By doing your own research about the school(s) you might attend, you can increase your likelihood of selecting a school that meets your current needs and expectations.

If you were working before you became disabled, you may

assume at first that you are unable to return to your previous job. In more cases than not, that assumption is inaccurate. Many jobs can be performed as well from a wheelchair as by an "able-bodied" employee. Some jobs may require modifications to the job site or a change in responsibilities, but many people will be able to return to their old positions with no change whatsoever or with minimal modifications. As a result of better laws about transportation and building accessibility and affirmative action programs that encourage employers to hire workers with disabilities, employment opportunities have been increasing steadily over the past decade. Whether you are returning to an old job or applying for a new one, the important thing is to be confident of what you *can do* while being realistic about those things you cannot do.

If something you cannot do seems to be an insurmountable obstacle, check with resources like the Paralyzed Veterans of America Advocacy Program, your state vocational rehabilitation office, or local independent living centers for information about ways to overcome what may at first appear to be an obstacle. Chances are that someone has faced a similar problem in the past and has come up with a solution.

Large employers often provide assistance to their current employees who become disabled, particularly if that disability was work-related. For work-related disabilities, employers are required to pay Workers' Compensation benefits if the employee is unable to return to work. Even if the injury was not work-related, it makes good economic sense for an employer to retain a current employee rather than to go to the expense of hiring and training a replacement. Employers also can obtain tax credits for making some modifications to jobs or jobs sites for the benefit of employees who become disabled, so there are solid economic reasons for an employer to want you back.

If you are unable to return to your old position because of your disability, or if you have not been in the workforce before becoming disabled, you may feel at a disadvantage by having to cope with job hunting and a new disability at the same time. However, knowing your strengths is the most important attribute you can have when looking for a job. What we perceive in ourselves to be disadvantages may be immaterial to prospective employers or may actually serve as an advantage if the employer is under pressure to hire "minorities," including people with disabilities. To assume that your disability is a disadvantage in an employment situation can be self-defeating.

Programs exist to aid persons with disabilities in becoming employable and in becoming employed. State vocational rehabilitation services assess clients for skills and functional ability and provide funding for job training, job site modifications, and purchase of equipment to assist you in performing your professional responsibilities. Every state has a Department of Vocational Rehabilitation, which is listed under state government offices in the telephone book. Contact your state agency for particular details about your state's program because each state has the freedom to develop its vocational rehabilitation program in a way most suitable for that state. Independent living centers also are good resources for information about employers in the community who are particularly supportive of workers with disabilities. A listing of some of these independent living centers can be found in Appendix 1.

The Veterans Administration provides vocational training for some veterans depending on the time of active duty and the severity of the disability. Contact your local office of the Veterans Administration or a PVA Service Officer for information about vocational education benefits available through the VA.

A spinal cord injury is not necessarily an impediment to employment. Other problems associated with the disability such as transportation, building accessibility, and attitudinal barriers—yours and your employer's—can be much more significant barriers, and resources exist for those who want to return to work. If education and employment are important to your life, those resources can be utilized to make the transition back to the workforce a little easier.

ADAPTIVE AIDS

Adaptive aids can play an important role in assisting you to adapt physically to an environment that was designed for people who are not disabled. Automotive adaptive equipment can provide a significant degree of independence that otherwise would not be possible. The standard method of driving an automobile involves the use of two hands and two feet. Automotive adaptive equipment allows you to use hand controls to brake and accelerate. Thus, most people with paraplegia and many with quadriplegia are able to drive a car or van with the addition of hand controls. In addition, a lift can be attached to a van, and the driver's seats can be removed so that you can drive a van without transferring out of the wheelchair.

Limited hand function can severely diminish the ability of a quadriplegic person to perform self-care, to write, or to operate light switches, television knobs, and thermostats. Several kinds of devices have been developed to aid quadriplegics in regaining the ability to perform those kinds of tasks. Some of these devices are modifications to the item that is to be operated; others are adaptive devices worn by the individual.

Occupational therapists often are good sources of information about adaptive equipment that is on the market, as well as about low-cost modifications that can be made by you or a member of your family to increase independence. We have listed some of the better resources on adaptive equipment in the "Suggested Readings" section at the end of this chapter. An additional resource for information about adaptive aids is NARIC, or the National Rehabilitation Information Center. NARIC is supported by the National Institute for Disability Research and Development (NIDRR) and is located on the grounds of Catholic University in Washington, D.C. NARIC maintains a computerized data base, ABLEDATA, which has product information on devices and systems for persons with disabilities. They can perform a search on devices and systems that may be useful to you. For information about their services, write to NARIC at 4407 8th Street, NE, Washington, DC 20017.

Occasionally an individual has a need for which no commercially available product can be found. In addition, improvements often are needed to existing products to make them more useful, and there are disability-related problems for which no products have yet been devised. Within the past two decades, a specialized field called *rehabilitation engineering* has developed to address the problem of device development for the needs of people with disabilities. Many rehabilitation centers now have a rehabilitation engineer or a rehabilitation engineering program to develop new products for their patients and clients in the community. Both the Veterans Administration's Rehabilitation Research and Development Service and NIDRR provide support for specially designated rehabilitation engineering centers, all of which have developed expertise in specific areas of rehabilitation engineering.

Both the VA and NIHR centers are good sources of information about devices that are available and about current research efforts. Addresses and phone numbers for each of these centers are listed in Appendix 1.

Any spinal cord injury is a severe disability, but the most severely disabled among the spinal cord–injured population are those with an injury at the C1 through C3 level because respiratory function and every other function below that level is affected. The question of how to provide appropriate assistance to respirator-dependent quadriplegics was not even asked until recent years, because few survived their initial injuries. But today that situation has changed as a result of improved emergency care and the development of new treatment techniques. Providing the medical care and support services for disabled individuals has become a major financial

and ethical issue for many facilities. Many rehabilitation facilities are equipped to handle only one or two such individuals
at a time; others simply do not accept patients with such severe disabilities. To find an appropriate facility for rehabilitation of a person who is respirator-dependent, first make contact with one of the Model Regional SCI Treatment Centers
or VA SCI Centers (Appendix 1).

Respirator dependency and the degree of disability associated with such an injury may lead one to believe that this
truly is an "unrehabilitatable" disability. Fortunately that is
not the case. Although the severity of the disability cannot be
minimized, this is one area in which technology truly is making
immense strides to overcome the otherwise devastating
effects.

Some people with high cervical lesions can be weaned from
the respirator for several hours at a time or even completely.
Phrenic nerve stimulators are being used in some individuals
to improve respiratory function. Other people may require
continuous assistance with respiration, but often such systems
can be made portable to allow for mobility.

Many people who are respirator-dependent are able to move
back into the community, provided they have assistance with
activities of daily living and the proper equipment to aid with
breathing and mobility.

Wheelchair accessories, such as reclining mechanisms,
portable respiration systems, environmental control units, and
postural supports, can help a severely disabled person become
more mobile and more independent. Essential to success,
however, is the presence of some sort of support system consisting either of family, friends, paid attendant care, or a combination of these. Rehabilitation facilities familiar with the
needs of respirator-dependent quadriplegics can assist these
individuals and their families in acquiring the necessary specialized equipment.

The needs and problems of people who are respirator-dependent are greater than those of most paraplegics and quad-

riplegics. Nevertheless, appropriate equipment, good medical care, and the development of a strong personal support system can do much to improve the quality of life for someone with such a severe disability.

SUMMARY

The transition from hospital to home can be simplified by careful planning while still in the hospital and by conducting a realistic evaluation of what your needs will be when you return home. If resources such as independent living centers, other disabled persons in the community, and rehabilitation center staff are used, the tensions associated with such a transition can be reduced significantly.

SUGGESTED READINGS

The Accessible Home: Remodeling Concerns for the Disabled (1981). Reprinted with permission from Better Homes and Gardens Remodeling Ideas, Copyright Meredith Corp. Available from Paralyzed Veterans of America, 801 Eighteenth St., N.W., Washington, DC 20006.

Access Information Bulletin. Available through Paralyzed Veterans of America, 801 Eighteenth St., N.W., Washington DC 20006.

Adaptive Environments Center (1981): *Environments for All Children.*

Barrier Free Environments, Inc. (1981): *Doors and Entrances.*

Barrier Free Environments, Inc. (1980): *Choosing an Accessibility Consultant.*

Barrier Free Environments, Inc. (1980, 1985): *Adaptable Housing.*

Bjerkesett, M. (1981): *Multi-Family Housing.*

Cochran, W. (1981): *Restrooms.*

Cotler, S. R. (1981): *Elevators and Lifts.*

Dibner, E. (1981): *Locating Accessible Facilities.*

Kiewel, H. D. (1981): *Ramps, Stairs and Floor Treatments.*

Leibrock, C., and Rowe, L. (1981): *Interior Furnishings and Space Planning.*

Levin, B., Paulson, R., and Klote, J. (1981): *Fire Safety.*

Orleans, P. (1981): *Kitchens.*

Orleans, P. (1981): *Single Family Housing Retrofit.*

Plourde, R. M. (1980, 1985): *Recreation.*

Ruddy, N. (1981): *ANSI A117.1 (1980) Survey/Checklist.*

Assistance for the Handicapped, A Directory for Federal and State Programs to Help the Handicapped to Employment. President's Committee on Employment of the Handicapped, 1111 20th St., N.W., Washington, DC 22036.

Breaking New Ground. Department of Agricultural Engineering, Purdue University, West Lafayette, IN 47907 (geared to disabled farmers).

Bruck, L. (1978): *Access: The Guide to a Better Life for Disabled Americans.* David Obst Books, Random House, New York NY.

Checklist of Income Tax Deductions for Medical Expenses. United Cerebral Palsy Association, Inc., Legal Dept., 66 East 34th St., New York, NY 10016.

Design of Bathrooms, Bathroom Fixtures and Controls for the Able-Bodied and Disabled (1980). Final Report. National Institute of Handicapped Research, U.S. Dept. of Education and College of Architecture and Urban Studies, and Virginia Polytechnic Institute and State University, Blacksburg, VA.

Directory of National Information Sources on Handicapping Conditions and Related Services (Order #0065-00-00142-0). U.S. Dept. of Education, Office of Special Education and Rehabilitative Services, Clearinghouse on the Handicapped, Washington, DC 20202.

Enrichments . . . Helping Hands for Special Needs. Enrichments Inc., P.O. Box 3340, Grand Rapids, MI 49501. (Products to promote independent living)

Equipment for the Disabled. The Disability Rights Center, Suite 1124, 1346 Connecticut Ave., N.W., Washington, DC 20036.

Fact Sheet on Handicapped Assistance Loans. U.S. Small Business Administration, 1111 18th St., Washington, DC 20416.

Free Guide to Home Health Care Products. Self-Care, Inc., 149 Marion Drive, Dept. B, West Orange, NJ 07052.

A Guide to Controls: Selection, Mounting, Applications. Rehabilitation Engineering Center of Children's Hospital at Stanford. Children's Hospital at Stanford, 520 Willow Rd., Palo Alto, CA 94304.

Hale, G. (ed.) (1981): *The Source Book for the Disabled.* Bantam Book, 666 Fifth Ave., New York, NY 10103.

In Search of Barrier Free Housing (May 1981). Reprinted with permission from *Paraplegia News.* Copyright Paralyzed Veterans of America.

Keralaguen, A.: *Clothing Designs for the Handicapped.* Accent Publications, P.O. Box 700, Bloomington, IL 61702.

Laurie, G.: *Housing and Home Services for the Disabled: Guidelines and Experiences in Independent Living.* Harper & Row Publishers, Inc., Medical Dept., 2350 Virginia Ave., Hagerstown, MD 21740.

503: A Law Meaning Job Rights for Handicapped People. Mainstream, Inc., 1200 15th St., N.W., Washington, DC 20005.

McGeough, C. S., Junjohan, B., and Thomas, J. L. (eds.) (19■■): *The Directory of College Facilities and Services for the Handicapped.* Oryx Press, 2214 North Central at Encanto, Phoenix, AZ 85004-1483.

Raschko, B. B. (1982): *Housing Interiors for the Disabled and Elderly*. Van Nostrand Reinhold, New York. Van Nostrand Reinhold Mail order Service, 7625 Empire Drive, Florence, KY 41042.

Rehabilitation Purchasing Guide, Rehabilitation Encyclopedia. Order from IMS Press, 426 Pennsylvania Ave., Fort Washington, PA 19034.

The Rights of Physically Handicapped People. American Civil Liberties Union, 132 W. 43rd St., New York, NY 10036.

Sargent, J. V.: *An Easier Way—Handbook for the Elderly and Handicapped*. Accent Publications, P.O. Box 700, Bloomington, IL 61702.

Sutherland, A. T. (1984): *Disabled We Stand*. Indiana University Press, 10th and Morton Streets, Bloomington, IN 47405.

151 Tax Deductions You Can Take. Accent Publications, Gillum Rd. and High Drive, P.O. Box 700, Bloomington, IL 61701.

Thomas, J. L., and Thomas, C. H. (eds.) (1981): *Academic Library Facilities and Services for the Handicapped*. Oryx Press, 2214 North Central at Encanto, Phoenix, AZ 85004.

CHAPTER 6

Getting on with Your Life

Peter Axelson

I sustained my spinal cord injury a decade ago. Not long afterwards I found that trying to live as I had lived before my injury was frustrating and slow. I simply could not continue to do the same activities as before—"normal life," by my old definition, was going to be impossible for me.

As I learned new ways to carry on in life, I began to analyze the kinds of activities I had most enjoyed before my injury. I tried to remember exactly what sensations, experiences, and feelings were associated with the various activities I had liked. In skiing, for example, my objective had never been simply to go down a hill on two feet. Rather the core experience had to do with the exhilaration of movement, the snow, the challenge to my skill, the beauty of the mountains, the wind in my face, the companionship of friends.

Normality for me was still the goal. But my objective was redefined: I would seek out activities—but with my basic personality, my basic drives. My life would be normal when I achieved a balance between mental, physical, and spiritual activity that reflected who I truly am—with or without a disability.

EXAMINING YOUR ACTIVITY LEVEL

In this chapter you will have the opportunity to examine your life before you were injured—how you lived and what

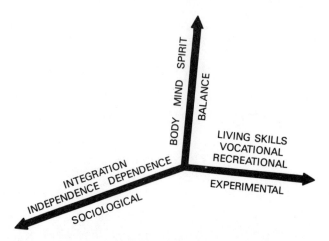

FIG. 6.1. Achieving balance in your life.

you cared about—and the importance this has for developing your present and future life. The purpose of the exercise below is to assist you to begin to take control of your life as it is now, through an objective assessment of your basic personality and drives.

In this chapter we will examine three basic dimensions in which all human beings live their lives (Fig. 6.1). These dimensions are the following:

1. *Everyday living.* How you balance your daily living, vocational, and recreational activities
2. *Personal balance.* Your unique balance of body, mind, and spirit
3. *Relationships.* Your interactions with others—dependence, independence, and interdependence

BALANCING EVERYDAY ACTIVITIES

First look back to the activities that you performed every day, day in and day out, before sustaining your spinal cord injury. Think about the kinds of things you used to do during a typical day. Then divide each of those activities into one of three categories: *daily living, vocational,* and *recreational activities*. It is not so important that you have a particular activity lumped into the "right" category as much as it is important to be consistent between the first and second parts of this exercise. For example, you might consider sleeping to be a daily living activity or a recreational activity. Either definition is fine, as long as you are consistent throughout the exercise. The purpose is not to compare yourself with any sort of norm, but to observe your past and present activities objectively.

Determine the percentage of time that you used to spend in each of the following activities. The hours you assign to each category should total 24.

How Your Time Was Spent Before Your Spinal Cord Injury

Daily living activities	_____
Vocational activities	_____
Recreational activities	_____
Total hours	24

Determine the relative importance of each of these types of activities for achieving a balanced lifestyle. Give each of these activities a priority score between 0 and 10 such that the total of priority scores equals 10.

Priorities Today

Daily living activities	_____
Vocational activities	_____
Recreational activities	_____
Total priority score	10

Determine Present Activity Patterns

Think about your activities over the last week. Determine the percentage of time which you spent doing each of these types of activities. The total should again come to 24 hours.

Time Spent Today

Daily living activities	_____
Recreational activities	_____
Vocational activities	_____
Total percentage of time	24 hours

INTERPRETING THE RESULTS

Compare the percentage of time that you spent in each of the activity patterns yesterday with the percentage of time you spent in each of the activity patterns before you were injured. If you are still living within a rehabilitation environment, chances are that you are spending a greater percentage of time on your daily living activities than you were before your disability. After all, your total focus at first is to regain control of the physical aspects of your life.

By reviewing the relative importance to you of each of those activities and by reflecting on the percentage of time that you are currently spending on each of the categories of activities, you may identify a direction to work toward, a workable balance that will feel more natural as your physical mastery increases.

After my injury, I found that I was spending a tremendous amount of time on my daily living activities. I couldn't imagine how I would be able to return to school full time when I was spending over an hour just to get dressed and attend to my personal hygiene. But within 2 months, the same tasks took me about 15 minutes. I slowly became freer to focus on other needs.

Within my rehabilitation center there were no activities that required or taught recreational skills. Yet before my injury I had been active in both team and individual sports. Since entertainment had never been a satisfying recreational outlet for me, it was important to communicate to therapists my desire to learn recreational skills that I could utilize after leaving the rehabilitation center.

I first addressed the problem by having a friend bring his kayak to the rehabilitation center. The therapists were co-operative in helping me experiment by using the kayak in the swimming pool, and I found it was indeed an appropriate rec-reational activity for me, given some modifications to the kayak and learning special handling techniques. My rehabi-litation center was quite willing to help me learn recreational skills when I requested it.

Once you have decided to create a new balance between the kinds of activity in your life, it is also important to *schedule* the time to achieve that balance. Having a spinal cord injury means that your daily physical requirements will simply re-quire more time. No matter how efficiently I set up my home, inevitably some very simple tasks—such as putting away the dishes after a meal—take longer (I have broken a few dishes while trying to disprove this fact). So it is extremely important to schedule your time for the recreational and vocational ac-tivities that are vital to your well-being.

YOUR PERSONALITY BALANCE

We are going to shift focus now. Instead of looking at your practical activities, let's look at the different dimensions of your personality as you function in daily living. The three ways in which one interacts with the world could be defined as follows:

Physical

This refers to the ways in which you physically or bodily interact with the world around you, including your focus on fulfilling basic physical needs (eating, sleeping, exercise, etc.).

Intellectual

This refers to the mental realm, how you use your reason-ing, logic, and imagination to engage in vocational activities, learning, reading, writing, and so on.

Spiritual

Here I refer to that portion of one's life that provides motivation and purpose to push forward, which may be nurtured through quiet reflection, introspection, writing in a journal, religious activity, communing with nature, etc.

THE BALANCE BETWEEN BODY, MIND, AND SPIRIT

Analyze the percentage of time that you used to spend in physical, intellectual, and spiritual activities. Try to imagine a typical day before your spinal cord injury and determine which activities or experiences within that day were primarily motivated by physical, intellectual, or spiritual needs. Remember that each person's definition of these needs may be different, and that certain activities may satisfy more than one kind of need. (In my case, for example, sailing fulfills all three.) Again, your recorded times for all three categories should total 24 hours.

Time Spent Before Injury

Physical activities	_____
Intellectual activities	_____
Spiritual activities	_____
Total	24 hours

Examining Your Priorities

What is the relative importance of physical, intellectual, and spiritual activity in your life? Rate each activity on a 0 to 10 scale. Your total for the three dimensions should be 10.

Priorities Today

Physical	_____
Intellectual	_____
Spiritual	_____
Total	10

CURRENT ACTIVITY BALANCE

Determine the percentage of time you now spend in activities that fulfill your physical, intellectual, and spiritual needs.

Time Spent Today

Physical activities	_____
Intellectual activities	_____
Spiritual activities	_____
Total	24 hours

Comparing the proportion of time you now spend on physical, intellectual, and spiritual activity to the balance that you had before your injury may help you pinpoint some goals for change or development of your present priorities.

ESTABLISHING OR REESTABLISHING BALANCE

Depending on the level of your spinal cord injury you may wonder how you are going to make any changes in the balance of your activity patterns based on what you can do now. If you are a physically oriented person and have a very high spinal cord injury, for example, chances are that the lack of physical activity is going to feel quite frustrating. You can try to deal with these frustrations intellectually and you can try to maintain a positive spirit and attitude until you are ready to crack. However, in this instance you are going to have to try and determine some means of physically expressing yourself or you are going to be fundamentally dissatisfied with your new life.

During my rehabilitation program a natural desire for such a balance led me to focus on a whole new part of myself. For one thing, I now had the time to do things I had rarely done before, and I found I liked them: writing poetry, keeping a journal, listening to music, working with my hands, playing backgammon.

One development of lasting importance for me was an increasing intellectual involvement in my own rehabilitation: I studied spinal cord injury, the drugs and therapies used, the neurological system, and how its functioning was changed by my injury. I also started to design adaptive sports equipment and that helped to serve my needs for both intellectual and physical challenge.

The more I learned, the more I was able to take control of my rehabilitation program by asking questions and being involved in making decisions. I did some reading to learn about the side effects of different drugs. I also learned, for example, that different drugs were available to treat a given bladder infection. I was able to tell my physician about the side effects that I was having and a different drug was prescribed for me. Before, I had not even known that there were options for treating an infection.

Accepting your disability does not mean relinquishing all control of your physical environment. Rather, through adaptive equipment and other people you can express and exert control over your physical environment. Actually, all technologies are designed to enable people to manipulate and exert control over their environment.

RELATIONSHIPS

The third dimension in this examination process is that of interdependence, your relationship with others. Here we will deal with three distinct qualities:

Independence

By independence I mean those activities which you perform independently from other people. Another definition of the term would be your attitude toward the environment around you. If you are in control of the situation or your environment, then you are viewed as being independent.

Dependence

The requirement to depend upon other people to perform a particular activity or to function in your daily life.

Interdependence

A combination of independence—control over your environment and activities—and dependence upon others.

EXAMINATION OF TYPICAL RELATIONSHIP PATTERNS

Determine the percentage of time that you used to spend before your spinal cord injury doing things independently, dependently, and interdependently. You will have to be the judge in determining which activities you will classify as independent or which you will classify as dependent and interdependent. The purpose of the exercise is not to compare yourself with other people or even to make correct determinations, but to compare your relationships and activities before your spinal cord injury to the balance that exists now.

Time Spent Before Injury

Independent	_____
Dependent	_____
Interdependent	_____
Total	24 hours

EXAMINATION OF PRIORITIES FOR INDEPENDENCE, DEPENDENCE, AND INTERDEPENDENCE

Determine the relative importance to you of performing activities dependently, independently, and interdependently on a scale of 0 to 10. Your total for all three should equal 10.

Priorities

Independent	_____
Dependent	_____
Interdependent	_____
Total	10

DETERMINE PRESENT RELATIONSHIP PATTERNS

Determine in your present situation how many hours daily you are now spending doing things independently, dependently, and interdependently.

Time Spent Today

Independent	_____
Dependent	_____
Interdependent	_____
Total	24 hours

Compare the percentage of time spent on independent, dependent, and interdependent activities before your spinal cord injury with your present situation. Given your fundamental attitude toward being independent of or dependent on other people, can you identify a need to increase or decrease your independence now?

Dependence as a way of functioning can mean security for one person and insecurity for another. One of the issues that arises early in the rehabilitation experience is that of dependence on others for even the simplest physical needs. You may need to acknowledge your feelings on this issue.

Dependence on devices, systems, and other people is usually a reality for people with spinal cord injuries. However, everyone needs choices and options. A person who has a choice between dependence and independence and chooses dependence will have a different attitude from the person who is not given the choice.

The issue of control arises when talking about independence. When you are in control of the situation or in control of your environment, you are viewed as being independent. A certain degree of independence is important but there is sometimes an overemphasis on independence in the rehabilitation environment.

Interdependence lies somewhere between dependence and independence. All human societies are based on interdependent relationships. More than most other people, however, to live an interdependent lifestyle the person with a disability must have the strength and courage to communicate openly with others when help is needed and when independent action is preferred.

REESTABLISHING BALANCE BETWEEN DEPENDENCE, INDEPENDENCE, AND INTERDEPENDENCE

Technology

By using adaptive equipment, people with spinal cord injuries can control their environments and perform daily living, vocational, and recreational tasks with a greater degree of independence. For example, a simple electronic home control system enables me to turn off the lights in my bedroom from the bed instead of from a wall switch. At night I can turn on all of the outside lights if I hear something outside. Hand controls for foot-operated equipment allow me to operate everything from an automobile to an industrial sewing machine. The personal computer enables even those people with high spinal cord injuries to write and to communicate with others through the modem.

When a device or system fails, the end result can be catastrophic. Running out of battery power in subzero weather or failure of environmental controls can result in situations that lead to everything from inconvenience to life-threatening conditions. I have always tried to take time to learn about adaptive equipment in a controlled environment with assistance from someone else so that I was not putting myself at risk. Determine what happens if the power fails or if the attachment points come loose. Try new tricks with help from others before doing them on your own.

Any device or system that makes life easier for most people will benefit people with spinal cord injuries. Keep in mind, though, that you can get carried away with efficiency measures. Individuals who decide to use devices and systems are setting themselves up to be dependent on those devices and systems. Many people desire to be independent of devices and systems and prefer to be dependent on other people.

People

Many people with spinal cord injuries depend on able-bodied attendants to enable them to perform daily living, vocational, and recreational activities. The assistance of a professional attendant may mean greater control over their environment and daily life activities. The degree of control that one achieves can be problematic if the attendant relationship is one of a personal nature. Your family may want to help you do things, for example, whereas what you may need most is help doing things for yourself. Communication is the key ingredient to making dependent relationships work.

Communication

It is extremely important to be able to express your feelings and needs to other people upon whom you may be relying for assistance. If you do not feel confident expressing your needs to another person, it will be difficult for you to ask for or receive help.

The same is true if you wish to refuse assistance. When you want to do something on your own it is important to inform other people around you who might wish to assist and aren't sure if they should help or not. It is difficult for most people to watch you do something when they feel that they can do it more quickly or easily. I recall an occasion at the airport. I was loading duffel bags (which are easier to manage in a wheelchair than traditional suitcases) into the front seat of my truck. I wanted to load everything in a small space so I could see out of the right-hand mirror. A man came by and asked if I needed help. I refused, thanking him for his offer. To my astonishment he grabbed one of my bags from the cart I had used to bring them out and started ramming it into the truck anyway. I had to repeat my refusal of assistance more force- fully and explain that I wished to load the bags on my own. I tried to explain to him that he should not help without being asked or without asking himself. I also explained that he should realize that just because he felt he could load the bags with less effort than I, this did not give him reason to do it anyway. Finally he understood and apologized. I must say, though, that it has taken me a long time to be direct when such incidents occur. This is particularly true with regard to the members of my own family, each of whom cared for me and tried to help me deal with my day-to-day coping with a disability. We learned that assistance is not always helpful if the helper feels obligated to help and never has the opportunity to say "no." I also learned that assistance was not always what I needed from my family, but it was the easiest thing to share. Feelings come, eventually.

Interdependence always means an exchange. That means that your relationships—like all human relationships—are re- ciprocal. Perhaps you have work skills or a business which could provide services in exchange for help from other people. When people close to you are just plain nice and help without asking for anything in return, tell them how much you appre- ciate that help and ask if there is some way that you can repay them or if there is something you can do for them. I have some friends who help out and refuse to ask for anything in return. For these special friends I try to find out what their hobbies and interests are so that I can purchase or do something for them in return for their assistance and support.

Often, the only appropriate compensation for assistance from another person is money. If money is being exchanged, be up front about asking what assistance or services you will be receiving and how much those services will cost.

Building New Relationships

Most of your needs for interaction with others will be unchanged by your injury, but a few needs may be new to you. They include the development of social and functional skills.

If you have a spinal injury, you are going to learn new social skills simply because people will react to your company in ways that are new to you. You will find that some people react more to your disability than to your self, and that some people react in inappropriate ways. Some of these reactions are amusing, others are not. Most wheelchair users can tell you stories of able-bodied people presuming them to be deaf, of salespeople who were surprised to discover they carried their own money, of others who behaved as if spinal injuries were horribly contagious, and of some to whom a person in a wheelchair simply did not exist. You will have to learn how to deal with these reactions.

You may feel intimidated (or angered) the first time someone starts talking to you loudly and slowly. Your reaction to their manner of speech may be as inappropriate as their reaction to your spinal cord injury. Unless you choose an occupation directly related to disability such as physical therapy, you are unlikely to associate with other people with disabilities in the workplace. These associations will most often be made in recreational activities, and they constitute an extremely valuable support system for you in learning to manage your disability. They certainly have served that function for me.

One advantage of associating with people who have disabilities similar to your own is that you will learn important skills from them. Just as schools cannot teach you everything you need to get along in the world, neither can a rehabilitation center. Traveling with other people with disabilities, such as a team of wheelchair athletes, taught me a great deal about mobility and other aspects of my new life. I learned things from my teammates that even the best-intentioned physical therapist without a disability is not qualified to teach. How do you get your suitcase out of the baggage carousel? How do you use an escalator? How do you get back from the salad bar without spilling food on your lap? (Which I still have not figured out.)

How do you hail a taxi? In a strange town, where can you get a cracked wheelchair frame rewelded, quickly and economically? These are all things that I learned after finishing my formal rehabilitation.

Participating in wheelchair sports taught me that I could laugh about my disability. I learned that the problems that I was having are the same problems that everyone in a wheelchair has.

SUMMARY

Having a disability does not change your basic human need for balanced activity. Your personality—those unique inner physical, intellectual, and spiritual traits that make up your "self"—remain much the same even though a spinal cord injury has dramatically altered the functioning of your body.

During rehabilitation your primary focus is to regain control of the physical aspects of your life. Beyond that, however, is the requirement to examine your life and decide consciously where you want to go from here. The goal will be to begin to reestablish a balance that will bring you long-term satisfaction.

SUGGESTED READINGS

Corbet, B. (1980): *Options: Spinal Cord Injury and the Future.* Available through National Spinal Cord Injury Association, 149 California St., Newton, MA 02158.

Marinelli, R. P., and Dell Orto, A. E. (eds.) (1984, 2nd ed.): *The Psychological and Social Impact of Physical Disability*. Springer Publishing Co., 200 Park Ave. So., New York, NY 10003.
Trieschmann, R. B. (1987): *Aging with a Disability*. Demos Publications, 150 E. 61st Street, New York, NY 10021.
Wright, B. A. (2nd ed.): *Physical Disability—A Psychosocial Approach*. Harper & Row Publishers, 10 E. 53rd St., New York, NY 10022.

CHAPTER 7

Keeping Yourself Healthy

Peter Axelson

Your reward as you work to achieve a new balance in activity and expression will be a sense of satisfaction, positive body image, and a positive outlook on life. The foundation upon which your new life will rest, however, will be your health and general fitness. In this chapter we will take a look at some guidelines for maintaining fitness and good nutrition. Here's where to start:

- *Act.* Be active and start doing things with your body, mind, and spirit. Cause things to start happening within your life.
- *Be creative.* Experiment with all aspects of your body's present strength and limitations.
- *Listen.* And watch for feedback from your body.

The discussion to follow will be based on these general principles. While each section emphasizes physical activity, I would stress the importance of being active intellectually and spiritually as well.

DEVELOP AN EXERCISE PROGRAM

Be active—exercise. It is very important to start doing something with the abilities you have now. Although it is true that you will not be able to exercise the way that you used to, it is vitally important to use whatever function you have.

You are probably aware of people without disabilities who suffer from a lack of physical activity. They tend toward obesity, heart disease, and other maladies. Inactivity is a common problem in our culture. Each weekend, thousands of American athletes play; other Americans watch them. Lots of them need exercise, and so do you.

You need exercise more than ever before: Exercise will be more difficult than ever before; you have more excuses not to exercise than ever before; and you probably will have less encouragement to exercise than ever before. To counter all these factors, you will need to rely on your own self-motivation. Finding recreational activities that stimulate you will make this motivation easier to find.

Despite our best intentions, most of us do not exercise enough because we find "exercising" to be dull and tedious. Sports and recreational activity can replace this tedium with a more emotional and intense level of participation. A person climbing a mountain, for example, is likely to be thinking about the challenge of the climb, the spectacle of the scenery, and the fellowship of other climbers. A person doing chin-ups is likely to be thinking about muscle fatigue and how much time the exercise is taking. These two people are getting similar exercise, but one is playing, and the other is working. The time and effort they expend will depend on how much they enjoy these activities. In short, develop an exercise program that you can work with today, even if you are flat on your back (or flat on your stomach). Use whatever muscles you can. This will speed the pace with which you can develop new skills for your daily living, vocational, and recreational activities. If your state of mind is such that you don't want to do anything anymore, try doing the exercises anyway. New vistas will open to you as you gain strength.

Later in your rehabilitation you can contact the National Handicapped Sports and Recreation Association. This organization sponsors fitness clinics and workout programs in many cities throughout the United States. Also you can participate in an exercise program for people without disabilities.

Here are some of the key features of an ongoing exercise program to help you maintain fitness after your spinal cord injury.

STRENGTHENING

It is extremely important to develop as much strength as possible in the muscles that you can control because you are going to be relying on whatever muscle activity you have left to compensate for those portions of your body that are paralyzed. Just as athletes strengthen specific muscle groups to maximize their function in a particular athletic activity, you must strengthen specific muscle groups to perform specific activities.

I remember the first time I transferred in and out of an automobile. It had taken me about 20 minutes to get myself into the car, using a slide board to transfer. The last thing I wanted to do was to get back out. While learning this new skill, I had depleted the strength of the muscles needed to transfer anywhere. Yet the next day the same maneuver took only 10 minutes—and now I don't even think about it when I get in and out of cars. I'm free to concentrate on other things.

AEROBIC CONDITIONING

The heart and lungs have particular needs which people with spinal injuries may find difficult to meet. Loss of sensation and/or motor control will reduce (or even eliminate) exercise of whatever muscle groups are affected. What is less obvious is that cardiovascular exercise will also be reduced.

The heart cannot be exercised directly but only through vigorously exercising other muscles. During exercise, all muscles demand increased blood circulation, and this demand is met by increased heartbeat. So although we have no conscious control of our heart rate, we can exercise our hearts by increasing the loads we put on various muscles.

The basic ingredient for an aerobics program is repetitoon and continuous exercise. Any exercise that causes your heart rate to increase for a period of 15 minutes or longer will strengthen your heart. Hand-cycling and swimming are two activities that I have enjoyed while obtaining excellent aerobic benefits. If those resources are not available to you, push-ups off the arm rests of the wheelchair can be a convenient and quick way to get aerobic exercise.

ENDURANCE

In addition to building strength and getting aerobic conditioning, physical endurance is one of the most important ingredients for reestablishing a balance in your daily living, vocational and recreational activities. Without it you will find it difficult to do the things that bring you the most satisfaction.

When I first returned to a university environment some time after my injury, I found myself feeling weak by the time I rolled back to my dormitory in the afternoon. At the same time, I started an exercise program which consisted of swimming 45 minutes per day 5 days per week. Within a short time I had gained enough endurance to take all my school activities in stride.

MOVEMENT AND ALTERNATIVE POSTURES

We have talked about conditioning to build strength and endurance. While it is important to establish routines to attend to basic physiological functions such as bowel and bladder management, breaking one's routine in other areas can be very helpful. Think about what you are doing with your body the rest of the time. Breaking your routines by standing and stretching, and alternative sitting postures can do a lot to improve overall health and well-being.

BREAKING ROUTINES

The position of various braces and supports should be altered to vary the places where such equipment might rub on the skin. Even clothing—if worn in the same manner and same spot over and over again—can cause early development of an abrasion or pressure sore. The attachment of urological equipment to the same position on the same leg day after day can lead to the development of a skin abrasion. For men, the attachment of a condom with the same taping pattern day after day can cause the development of a pressure sore. In summary, think about how you can vary your daily routines— just enough to prevent abrasions or sores from developing.

STRETCHING

It is extremely important to move the joints of paralyzed extremities through their full range of motion and to stretch all the muscle groups affecting each joint. Doing so improves circulation and prevents contracture of your joints. One of the most important ways to stretch is standing, discussed below. I often perform stretching exercises after getting in bed at night.

STANDING

Standing has significant physiological, psychological, vocational, and recreational benefits. Physically, standing helps to strengthen the heart by requiring it to pump harder and improves circulation throughout the body. Standing puts the internal organs in proper alignment which improves respiratory and digestive function; it allows all urine to drain from the bladder (which is impossible in the sitting position) thus helping to prevent urinary tract infections. Standing stretches the muscles of the legs and back, and relieves pressure, temperature, and humidity at sitting surfaces. Evidence shows that standing also helps to prevent soft-tissue ossification (formation of calcium deposits in soft muscle tissue) and kidney stones.

When you first stand in the rehabilitation center you may be placed on a tilt platform. This is to bring you gradually to a standing position so that the sudden demand on your heart to pump the blood in a vertical direction does not cause lightheadedness or fainting.

The psychological benefits of standing are great. With a "standing wheelchair" you can have access to the environment and eye contact at the same level as other people. Recreational opportunities, such as dancing, archery, darts, golf, and cooking are enhanced in the standing position. So are

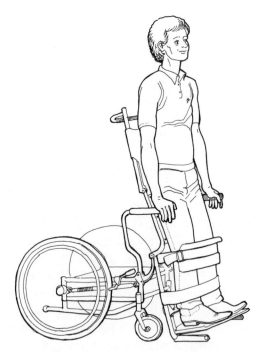

FIG. 7.1. Stand-up wheelchair.

vocational opportunities—a surgeon returned to work and began performing operations again soon after acquiring a wheelchair that allowed him to stand.

A standing wheelchair is now available which allows the user of the chair to stand at any time (Fig. 7.1). I have used such a wheelchair and find that it enhances my activities within the home environment. I recommend standing for at least 20 minutes a day. I myself use the time to catch up on my reading, and in fact I wrote many portions of this chapter while standing.

SITTING

Like most people with spinal cord injuries who find themselves sitting for greater portions of their lives, you know the importance of selecting a proper cushion for sitting. Equally important, though, is your sitting posture. When trying to position yourself in your wheelchair either by yourself or with assistance, work first at getting your pelvis centered in the middle of your cushion and level side to side. Then position your upper body. Try a small pad behind your lower back for lumbar support, then adjust your foot support(s) so that there is weight beneath your thighs. Experiment with adjusting the armrests if possible. If you need them, tape on a support for the arms or upper torso to determine if it is comfortable. Your wheelchair may soon look very strange, but you will have determined what works best. You can then go to a rehabilitation engineering center to have permanent modifications made which are visually more appealing.

Lie down whenever possible, roll over and let the blood circulate through the tissues in the buttock area. This will allow fabric in your clothing to cool off and will reduce humidity at the seating interface. If laying down is just not possible, move around in your wheelchair in addition to performing pressure releases as frequently as possible. Try moving yourself from side to side in your chair. Twist slightly left and right occasionally. Rocking or leaning your body forward and backward, and side to side, will cause a shift in your weight distribution at the seating interface. This will help to prevent pressure sores from developing.

Try to put your feet in a different position every so often. I have found that putting my feet on the floor off to the side of the front casters of my wheelchair puts more weight on my thighs and feet and less on my buttocks. Always make sure that the footrests are adjusted so that as much weight as possible is borne by the feet and thighs. This will reduce pressure to the buttocks.

FEEDBACK MECHANISMS

Your body is remarkably good at giving you information about its condition. The more carefully you listen to it, the healthier you will stay. For people with disabilities, prevention is the name of the game. For example, tiredness might be an indication that you need to take a break and get a breath of fresh air. However, if you have been pushing yourself for a long time, it might be time to get some rest. On the other hand, a headache, sore muscles, or weakness might be a sign that a low-grade bladder infection is developing—something that should be dealt with right away by having a urine culture performed.

Listen to your body, make changes and experiment, and note if the changes help any of the symptoms you're feeling. Don't forget to watch your body as well. Keep an eye on your body's excrement—texture, color, substance, etc.—and keep in touch with how your diet might be affecting your bowel management program. I like to keep an eye on my urine. The color and cloudiness of the urine may change throughout the day and this is an important pattern to recognize. Should a change in the pattern occur, I notice it right away.

BIOFEEDBACK TRAINING

Biofeedback is a treatment technique in which people are trained to improve their health in response to signals from their own body. You have used biofeedback when responding to the information given you by a simple thermometer or a bathroom scale. More sophisticated biofeedback techniques can help you relieve tension and pain, high and low blood pressure, and disorders of the digestive system—all symptoms which sometimes plague people with spinal cord injuries.

Biofeedback operates on a fairly simple principle. Special machines monitor the state of your internal bodily functions and give you feedback in the form of light or sound. One machine, for example, picks up electrical signals in the muscles. It activates an audible tone that increases as muscles grow more tense. If you want to relax the tension in those muscles, you work to lower the pitch of the tone. After a time, you learn to make the internal adjustments which will result in muscle relaxation, lowered blood pressure, reduced pain, and so on.

Biofeedback training has enabled me to learn to reduce tension and send a wave of relaxation throughout my body. Once I completed the training, I was able to perform the relaxation technique in any environment at any time without the biofeedback equipment. You may wish to contact a clinician or a psychologist working within a local rehabilitation center to inquire about learning and using biofeedback techniques.

WEIGHT

Weight is an important consideration for the person with spinal cord injury. Research has shown that atrophy occurs in the muscle tissue of paralyzed extremities; this atrophied tissue is often replaced with fat.

The percentage of ordinary body fat of a person with spinal

cord injury averages 20 to 25 percent while in most people 15 percent body fat is normal. This can be true even if the individual does not look obese but is the same weight as before acquiring the disability.

An ideal weight for most people with thoracic spinal cord injuries would be, on the average, 10 to 15 percent less than that recommended by standard tables of height and weight. The excess body weight makes it more difficult to perform the tasks associated with daily living, such as transfers, and increases the potential for pressure sores.

As with everyone else, if your percentage of ordinary fat is higher, the heart has to work harder to push blood through the smaller capillaries of fat tissue. This, in turn, will cause a greater susceptibility to diseases associated with the obesity— including a tendency to die earlier from heart disease.

SENSORY INPUT

Owing to the loss of sensation in lower extremities it is important to be attuned to the environment using the senses that you do have. If you have sensation in the hands, you can use them to feel the areas near your feet or legs for temperature. If you do not have sensation in any of your extremities, your mental alertness is critical for analyzing a situation for external hazards.

Those hazards could include the bending or breaking of bones in any of your extremities, or injury due to heat or cold. Paralyzed limbs, for example, do not sweat when the body heats up, so the body has a hard time cooling off. On the other hand, in very cold conditions the arteries will not constrict to prevent heat loss and maintain a stable body temperature.

EXPRESSIVE THERAPY

It is often said that your other senses become more acute when you are deprived of the use of one sense. "Expressive therapies'' using music, art, and dance can help you develop your present capabilities and become more attuned and responsive to your environment.

Expressive therapy is a holistic approach to diet, exercise, stress, or lifestyle change which combines the creative arts with more traditional therapies to release the potential in each person for movement and creative expression. A fairly new entry into the arena of available self-development techniques, it nevertheless shows promise for people with spinal cord injuries in developing awareness or skills to compensate for the disability.

Areas particularly addressed through expressive therapy include pain management and stress reduction, eating habits and diet, healing, problem solving, movement, and creative expression.

DIET AND NUTRITION

This section examines some basic tenets of good diet and nutrition, an issue which is particularly important for people with disabilities. What you put into your body will determine your ability to maintain health and fitness over the long term.

Dietary Considerations

The U.S. Department of Health and Human Services has issued some general and commonsense guidelines for maintaining a healthy diet. While these guidelines are applicable to everyone, I feel that they are especially important if one has a disability.

1. Eat a variety of foods—from fruits and vegetables, dairy products, and whole grains, to poultry, fish, and legumes (Fig. 7.2).
2. Maintain ideal weight. People with disabilities are like everyone else, in that obesity is dangerous to their health.

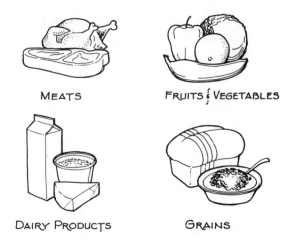

MEATS   FRUITS & VEGETABLES

DAIRY PRODUCTS   GRAINS

FIG. 7.2. Four basic food groups.

There is only one way to lose weight, and that is to eat less and increase physical activity.

3. Avoid too much fat and cholesterol. A high blood cholesterol level can lead to serious health problems, with a greater risk of heart disease.
4. Eat foods with adequate starch and fiber. Foods such as whole grain breads and cereals, fruits and vegetables, beans, peas, and nuts are good complex carbohydrates which help prevent bowel problems and provide energy for the body's needs.
5. Avoid too much sugar. Sugar causes tooth decay, can upset your blood sugar level, and provides calories without adding any nutrients to the diet.
6. Avoid too much salt. Sodium is an essential element for the body but in excess it leads to high blood pressure.
7. If you drink alcohol, do so in moderation. Alcohol is high in calories and reduces the absorption of vital nutrients by the body if taken in quantity.

I would also recommend that you eat as little red meat as

possible. It takes longer to digest and may cause constipation for those who are sedentary.

Water

By far the most important but overlooked ingredient in our diet is water; yet the intake of water is often never even discussed in relation to diet. A steady intake of water—at least 2½ to 3 quarts daily—is essential for the body to process other foods, fluids, and body wastes. With your doctor's consent, you can increase the volume of your urine by increasing your water intake, and this will decrease the mineral concentration in your kidneys and reduce the likelihood of kidney stone formation.

Monitoring Blood Sugar Level

For people who have trouble processing sugars—those who are either hypoglycemic or those who are hyperglycemic (diabetic)—it is important to monitor the intake of all foods to determine their effect upon blood sugar level. The effects of large sugar intake can be monitored on an informal basis. If you find that your energy level and moods swing dramatically, a pattern that coincides with eating meals, you may be somewhat hypoglycemic. Try to eat a small portion of protein (such as a small piece of cheese) between your regular meals, and limit your intake of simple sugars (fruit juices, soft drinks, candy, jelly, jam, etc.) at all times. If you suspect that you are hyperglycemic or hypoglycemic, it is possible to obtain a test for these conditions at a rehabilitation center or hospital. You can then take appropriate medication if necessary.

Types of Food

The majority of people with spinal cord injuries are constantly sitting and it is important to recognize how this affects the digestion of foods. Constant sitting causes the colon and bowels to be twisted or compressed compared with what they would be in the standing position. If you have irregular eating habits, are eating the wrong kinds of food and getting little exercise, your likelihood of having problems with constipation or irregularity are greatly increased.

I have found that my body has difficulty processing extremely rich foods, such as thick sauces and heavy desserts. In addition, eating red meat causes extreme discomfort in my bowels. It slows down my whole digestive system and causes a backup in my bowel program.

Constipation—a common problem among people with spinal cord injuries—can often be alleviated through a high fiber diet combined with ample fluid intake. At least four servings from the "grain group," and fruits and vegetables, should provide plenty of fiber to maintain a healthy bowel program without the continual use of laxatives and enemas (see more on this subject in Chapter 9).

MEDICATIONS

A medication is a substance that is taken to prevent or cure a medical problem. For a person with spinal cord injury, knowledge about and attention to the medications you are taking is important for overall management of your disability.

Be sure to write down and remember the information your doctor provides about the medications you are taking. You should know:

1. the name, purpose, and possible side effects of the medication;
2. dosage, storage (should it be refrigerated?), and timing for taking it;
3. any special precautions to remember (can it be combined with other medications? with alcohol? with food or dairy products?).

Some common medications used for treatment of persons with spinal cord injuries include the following:

Anticholinergics decrease the muscle activity of internal organs, especially the bowel and bladder.

Antibiotics fight infection by destroying the bacteria that cause it.

Antidiarrheal medication relieves diarrhea by decreasing the activity of the intestines.

Antispasticity medications relieve spasms of the skeletal muscles.

Didronel inhibits the deposits of calcium in the bones.

Hyperreflexia medications help decrease the blood pressure associated with automatic hyperreflexia.

Laxatives increase movement of the intestines to promote bowel evacuation.

Stool softeners help waste move through the intestines.

Important: Be sure to inform your health care professional about all medications you are taking, even nonprescription ones such as aspirins, laxatives, or antacids. Some drugs, when taken in combination with other drugs, can cause a serious reaction whether these are two prescription medications or a prescribed drug combined with a "recreational drug." And watch for allergic reactions, such as a rash, when you take medication. If such a reaction develops, stop taking the medication immediately and call your doctor.

When purchasing prescription medications, be sure to find out about the *generic* name as well as brand name of the drug. You may be able to save money by buying the medication under its generic name.

ANTIBIOTICS

If your doctor prescribes antibiotics for treatment of an infection, be sure to ask about any restrictions associated with the antibiotic. Be alert to any symptoms or side effects, such as a rash or headache. Antibiotics are designed to attack infectious organisms but unfortunately can attack beneficial organisms as well. A little bit of research and experimentation should enable you to determine how you can replace the beneficial organisms through your diet. Be sure to take all the medication prescribed by your doctor.

RECREATIONAL, STREET DRUGS, AND ALCOHOL

Mind-altering substances—such as pain killers and all recreational drugs including alcohol—have the potential to wreak havoc on a basic health maintenance program. This is simply because they may dull your awareness of early symptoms of problems in basic bowel, bladder, and skin care management. When a "street drug" (cocaine or amphetamines, for example) is used in combination with a prescribed medication the potential exists for a serious reaction, such as increased heart rate, blurred vision, or excessive sedation.

Alcohol also can cause serious medical complications when combined with several common drugs, including medications especially used to treat spinal cord injuries. Alcohol increases the sedative effect of antispasticity medications, hypnotics, anticholinergics, and sedatives like Darvon, and can lead to breathing problems and extreme drowsiness when used in combination with these drugs. Be sure to ask your doctor if you can take your medications in combination with alcohol.

PAIN MANAGEMENT

Little is known about the cause or incidence of phantom pain in people with spinal cord injury. Research indicates that anywhere from 25 to 75 percent of people with spinal cord injury suffer from phantom pain as a result of their paralysis.

Mechanisms for dealing with pain are many and varied (see Chapter 11). As a last resort, surgical procedures which may or may not lessen the pain are an option. Pain killers are another option, but they have side effects—the worst of which is that they can be habit-forming.

As I discussed earlier, biofeedback has been my most effective treatment for phantom pain over the long term. I use it almost exclusively in dealing with this problem.

CONCLUSION

This chapter has been most difficult for me to write, because I am not an "expert" in nutrition or medications. Yet the subject of diet, exercise, and overall wellness has been very important to me since my injury. Having a spinal cord injury does not make one "sick," and that is something society as a whole tends to overlook. I believe that, for those of us with spinal cord injuries, our ability to lead a balanced, productive life depends on our careful attention to the basics of personal health care.

You will find that proper diet and exercise will reward you in everything else you do, enhancing every aspect of your daily life. So listen to your body and pay close attention to its needs. In return it will help you use your physical, intellectual, and spiritual assets to the fullest.

SUGGESTED READINGS

Interrelationships of dietary and pharmacy services in nutrition support (1983). *Report of the Fourth Ross Roundtable on Medical Issues.* Ross Laboratories, Columbus, OH 43216.

Marshall, D., Rabold, J., and Wilson, E. (1983): *Staying Healthy Without Medicine.* Nelson-Hall, Inc. Publishers, 111 North Canal St., Chicago, IL 60606.

McGill, M., and Pye, O. (1978): *The No-Nonsense Guide to Food and Nutrition.* Butterick Publishing, New York.

Nutrition and Your Health—Dietary Guidelines for Americans (Pamphlet #656A, 1980). Dept. of Health and Human Services/USDA, Consumer Information Center, Pueblo, CO 81009.

United States Pharmacopeial Convention Dispensing Information (USPDI)—Advice for the Patient, Vol II (1983). Order through United States Pharmacopeial Convention, Inc., 12601 Twinbrook Parkway, Rockville, MD 20852.

CHAPTER 8

Urinary Function

Mark N. Ozer

One of the major consequences of spinal cord injury is interruption of the body's natural mechanisms for getting rid of wastes. Urination and bowel function (which will be discussed in Chapter 9) are functions that many of us take for granted unless we experience problems with them.

When a spinal cord injury occurs, the mechanisms that once controlled these vital bodily functions no longer work as they did prior to injury. Consequently, you will need to develop new methods of carrying out these functions in order to maintain overall health.

HOW THE SYSTEM WORKS

The urinary system has three major functions: the *formation* of urine—the job of the kidneys; the *storage* of urine so it can be excreted when appropriate—the job of the bladder; and the actual *excretion* of urine—the job of the muscles (detrusors) that control the action of the bladder and the muscles (sphincters) that lead from the bladder to the outside of the body via the *urethra* (Figs. 8.1 and 8.2)

The kidneys collect waste products that are filtered through an elaborate system of coiled tubes (nephrons) within the kidneys. As blood flows through this filtering process, waste products are removed and diluted with water to become urine. The ureters carry the urine from the kidneys to the bladder,

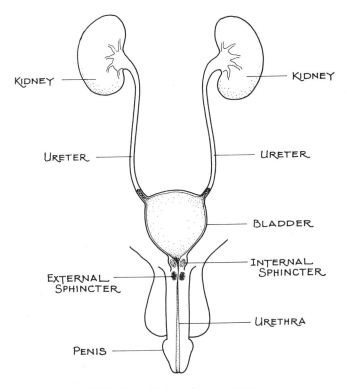

FIG. 8.1. Male urinary system.

which serves as a temporary storage place for urine. When the urine level in the bladder reaches a certain level, one experiences a sense of fullness that signals a need to urinate.

The actual act of urination requires coordination of several different actions simultaneously, all of which are coordinated at the *sacral level* of the spinal cord (Fig. 8.3). When you are ready to urinate, the sphincter controlling the flow of urine opens and the bladder contracts to expel its contents.

Immediately after a spinal cord injury occurs, the body goes into "spinal shock," during which many body systems shut down or cease to work properly. Although the person with an injury to the spinal cord may continue to produce urine in the

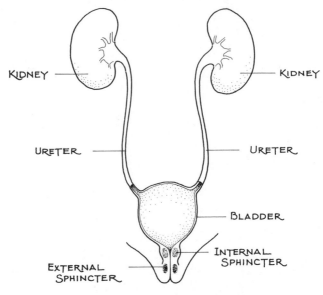

FIG. 8.2. Female urinary system.

kidneys, and the bladder continues to store the urine, the effect of the injury on the process of emptying the bladder is immediate. The bladder gets filled and cannot empty on its own.

The goals of early medical management of spinal cord injury are to prevent overdistension (stretching) of the bladder while also limiting the likelihood of infection. If the bladder becomes too distended (more than 500 cc) the muscles in its wall lose their elasticity and their ability to contract and empty. These muscles must be able to work again and they must be protected during this early period of spinal shock.

One traditional approach to emptying the bladder in the early period after spinal cord injury has been to use an indwelling catheter to prevent overdistention of the bladder. While an indwelling catheter may achieve that goal, a catheter can cause irritation to the bladder even if changed frequently and irrigated, and can lead to infection. Drainage of the blad-

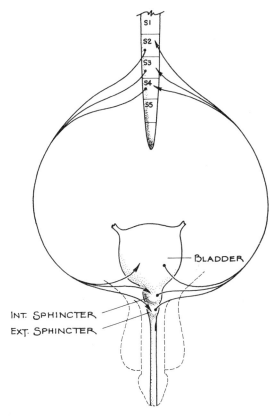

FIG. 8.3. Urinary function is controlled at the sacral level of the spinal cord.

der from the start with an indwelling catheter also can lead later on to a small bladder that will leak urine even if one continues to use an indwelling catheter.

The more common approach of bladder management immediately after injury today is *intermittent catheterization,* by which a catheter is inserted into the bladder at regularly scheduled intervals so that the bladder can be emptied but does not get too small or as easily infected.

BLADDER FUNCTION AFTER SCI

Once spinal shock wears off, you and your rehabilitation team will be able to determine how much and what kind of urinary function you will have.

Although the formation of urine in the person with spinal cord injury is generally the same as before injury, the bladder's function as a storage area is significantly altered. The urinary system is designed so that when your bladder is full, you will feel the urge to urinate and then empty the bladder. After a spinal cord injury occurs, the signal to urinate may be different from what it was before injury, or may be nonexistent. For many people, then, the clock replaces the body's warning system and the bladder must be emptied on a regular schedule to avoid back-up of urine.

The degree to which the process of excretion of urine is affected will vary depending on the level of injury and the sex of the person. Just as muscles to move arms and legs are affected differently depending on the level of the injury, so there are differences in the way the act of urination occurs.

The act of urination needs coordination of several different actions taking place simultaneously. The sphincters that control the flow of urine must open and the bladder must contract to expel its contents at the right time and place. This coordinated function usually is affected by damage to the spinal cord and in medical terms is called *dyssynergia*.

Sometimes the bladder does its job of contraction but the sphincter does not relax at the same time, or it may relax for only part of the time that the bladder is contracting. These conditions can be serious because urine tends to build up within the bladder.

DEVELOPING A BLADDER MANAGEMENT PROGRAM

Bladder control was achieved before your injury by nerves transmitting messages to and from the brain. When the bladder needed emptying, a message was sent warning you that your bladder was full. At that point you had a sensation of fullness and the need to urinate. If it was not convenient to do so, your brain sent a message through the spinal cord ordering the sphincter to tighten and the bladder to relax. With those messages received and acted upon, you were able to delay urination until a more convenient time. After you had arrived at a convenient time and place, the brain sent reverse messages, the bladder contracted, and the muscles in the external sphincter relaxed which opened to allow the urine to pass through.

After a spinal cord injury has occurred, the signals that indicated fullness and a need to void no longer are received by the brain. Consequently, the basic idea of a bladder management program is to develop a system to empty your bladder fully at regular intervals to avoid the serious complications that can occur as a result of urinary dysfunction, such as bladder or kidney stones, urinary tract infections, and kidney failure.

EVALUATION OF URINARY FUNCTION

People who have had spinal cord injuries usually undergo a number of tests to determine urinary function after injury. These tests help to determine what function you have retained, possible problems that you may encounter, and what kind of bladder management program is most appropriate for you. Tests that often are done in a urinary evaluation include:

- *Intravenous pyelogram* (IVP). An IVP is an X-ray of the kidneys that indicates how well your kidneys are functioning and whether or not any structural changes have occurred that could indicate possible kidney damage.
- *Cystoscopy*. A cystoscopy determines how well the bladder is emptying and whether there are any stones or infections present. A *cystoscope* is inserted into the

bladder so that the urologist, a physician who specializes in the urinary system, can look directly at the bladder internally.

- *Voiding cystourethrogram (VCU)*. A VCU is an X-ray of the bladder that is done while voiding to observe urinary function during voiding.
- *Cystogram*. A cystogram is an X-ray of the bladder.
- *Urodynamic studies*. Measurement of pressures in the bladder and urethras after filling occurs, and measurement of the muscle action of the sphincters in coordination with emptying.

BLADDER MANAGEMENT

Development of an appropriate bladder management program is essential to your health. Urinary tract infections and kidney stones are a common *but preventable* complication in many people with spinal cord injuries. Good bladder management is the first step toward preventing those complications. And, as we will discuss later, recognizing the signs of bladder and kidney dysfunction before the problem gets too severe is the second step toward ensuring a healthy urinary system.

The body's natural approach to bladder management is to "tell" you that it is time to void by providing you with a feeling of fullness or uncomfortableness in the abdomen when the bladder is full. Prompt and regular voiding is important for several reasons. First, voiding regularly helps to keep the bladder from becoming stretched or distended so that the muscles of the bladder do not lose their ability to expand and contract. Second, if the bladder gets too full, urine will back up into the ureters and kidneys (*reflux*), which can cause damage to those parts of the urinary system. Third, urine contains many bacteria which, if expelled regularly, do not create a problem. If, however, they are given a warm, moist place to grow (such as the bladder) they are likely to cause infections. Urine also contains little crystals and salts that under normal conditions are passed as you void. If they are allowed to stay in the bladder or kidneys, though, they tend to attach themselves to one another and cause bladder or kidney stones.

Consequently, one of the most important health-related issues in the period following a spinal cord injury is to develop a bladder management program that will do the job that your urinary system did automatically prior to your injury—void regularly and completely to minimize the risk of urinary tract complications. An additional goal will be to ensure that such a program interferes as little as possible with your daily lifestyle.

There are three major approaches to bladder management that are used by people with spinal injuries: (1) *catheter-free voiding,* (2) *intermittent catheterization,* and (3) use of an *indwelling catheter.* The type of approach you use (or a combination of approaches) will depend upon the level and severity of your injury and, therefore, upon what you are able to do without assistance.

Once spinal shock dissipates, you may be able to develop *reflex voiding,* in which the bladder is able to contract and thus assist you in controlling your voiding, even though you will not feel the sensation of fullness that signals the need to urinate. If your spinal injury is in the region of the sacral cord, the level that controls urination, you will have what is called a *hypotonic bladder.* In such a situation, the muscles in the bladder wall generally are not able to contract automatically to the degree necessary to empty the bladder.

The techniques used to empty the bladder vary from one person to another. Some people are able to stimulate voiding by tapping rhythmically with their fingers in the area of the bladder. Others can stimulate voiding by stroking their thighs, pulling on their pubic hairs, or digitally stimulating the rectum. *Créde,* pressing the abdomen to induce voiding, is another method you may wish to try.

Even if you are able to accomplish reflex voiding, it is likely that you will need to wear some kind of protection against

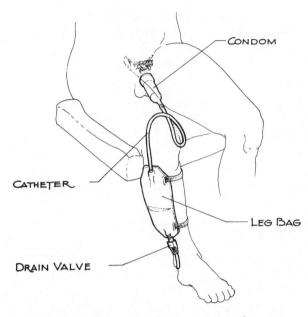

FIG. 8.4. External collection system for men.

involuntary leakage from the bladder. Many men wear a condom catheter, also referred to at times as an external catheter, external urinary collection device, "Texas catheter," or "gizmo." These are attached to a drainage bag that usually is strapped to the leg for ease of maneuvering (Fig. 8.4).

Women at this time do not have many options available for external urinary collection. While some female external collection devices have been developed and, in fact, are on the market, a woman with a spinal cord injury should be cautious about using them since the lack of sensation in the genital area could mask developing skin irritation. However, if your leakage problem appears to be slight, external pads (similar to large sanitary napkins) or diaperlike pads can be used to avoid wearing an internal catheter. Up-to-date information about urinary incontinence and ways to address this problem can be obtained by writing to Help for Incontinent People (HIP, Inc.), whose address is listed at the end of this chapter. Leakage problems for men and women alike also can be alleviated through the use of medications. Make sure you consult with your physician concerning the various options available for controlling urinary leakage.

INTERMITTENT CATHETERIZATION (IC)

Intermittent catheterization is a process by which a catheter is inserted into the bladder four or five times a day to drain the bladder of urine. One of the goals of intermittent catheterization is to promote *sterile urine*, i.e., urine that does not contain harmful bacteria. Another goal is to ensure that the bladder maintains its muscle tone. Consequently, intermittent catheterization will include a careful monitoring of how much liquid you take in and how much you excrete when you catheterize yourself. Normal bladder capacity is approximately 500 cc (about 1 pint).

During the rehabilitation phase, most people who are able to use intermittent catheterization will be taught how to perform the process for themselves. If you do not have sufficient hand function, a family member or nurse may do it for you. Generally, hospitals and rehabilitation centers use a *sterile technique*, whereby all equipment is sterile and sterile gloves are used to perform the procedure. However, many facilities now are teaching their patients to use a *clean technique* (i.e., does not require sterile equipment) when returning home. Your physician will be able to help you decide which approach is best for you.

INDWELLING CATHETERS

Some people with spinal cord injuries are unable to void without a catheter or to use intermittent catheterization. In order to ensure adequate urinary drainage, you then will need to use an *indwelling catheter* which you can leave in place as long as 3 or 4 months, if the catheter is draining well. However, it is important to clean the catheter twice a day for general hygiene and to eliminate places where bacteria can grow. Indwelling catheters are attached to a drainage bag that either is attached to your bed (when you are in the hospital) or to your leg when you are up and around.

Two types of indwelling catheters are used: those that are inserted through the urethral opening into the bladder; and those that are inserted into the bladder via an abdominal incision, called a *suprapubic catheter* or *ostomy*.

Sometimes, medications or surgery may be necessary to achieve a desired result. Some medications such as phenoxybenzamine promote urination by decreasing the contractions of the bladder neck. Surgery is occasionally used to relax the sphincters or to create a suprapubic opening for urinary drainage. If your medical treatment team recommends the use of medications or surgery to assist in bladder management, make sure you understand why this alternative has been recommended and what the pros and cons of that approach might be. Medications can have side effects or can interact inappropriately with other medications if medication use is not coordinated. Surgical procedures, too, can have side effects that should be explained to you thoroughly before you undergo them.

The type of urinary drainage system you will use will depend on many factors. Frank discussion with your rehabilitation team and others who have had spinal cord injuries will provide you with the best possible information about which alternative would be most appropriate for you to promote overall health.

AVOIDING PROBLEMS

The first goal in self-management is to prevent any infection of the urinary tract. The next goal is, if infection is present, to prevent illness and avoid being confined to bed or hospital.

Infection, once it gets started, must be treated as early as possible, both to prevent it from spreading throughout your body and to protect your kidneys. When a part of the kidney is destroyed, it can never be repaired. Thus the third goal is to get help when needed.

For most persons with spinal cord injury there are bacteria living in the bladder. It is important to keep these bacteria from multiplying to the point where they are enough to do damage. One way is to keep the bladder flushed so that urine does not stagnate and thus give bacteria a chance to multiply. One method easily available is to keep the urinary output high enough—generally in the range of 2 to 3 quarts (2000 to 3000 cc) each 24 hours.

The amount of residual urine left after you have emptied the bladder in your usual way is another important measure. You would check the amount remaining by catheterizing yourself. Watch for any increase, and check as often as is necessary for you. Some people find once a month about right, but you may need to check more or less often.

Measure the pH, or degree of acidity, of your urine as often as necessary. Healthy urine usually has a pH between 5 and 6. Bacteria, particularly those that can cause a chemical reaction with urea—one of the major waste products carried out in the urine—can raise the pH to the range of 8 or even higher, levels at which kidney or bladder stones are more likely to form.

Whether SCI patients should take medications that help maintain the acid level is a matter of some controversy; even more controversial is which medications work and how much to take. The issue is that the pH is a measure of the health of the urine, and when one monitors it, as a person with diabetes learns to monitor his urine for sugar, it becomes a sensitive measurement that can be useful for you in evaluating your own health.

The more frequently you monitor your kidney function the

more effective that management will be, and responding to early warning signals is most important.

Antibiotics are a group of medications that help slow down the rate at which bacteria multiply so that the body's defenses, the white blood cells that fight infection, can catch up and prevent the bacteria from killing more tissue. Antibiotics help to control infections of the kidneys as well as prevent infections from spreading to the rest of the body. It is important to understand that many antibiotics that act in the urine do not destroy bacteria but only slow down the rate of growth. This group of antibiotics are called *bacteriostatic*, that is, they keep the number of bacteria "static." Although antibiotics are important, they can't do the job by themselves. To get the best results with the fewest side effects, medications must be used early in the onset of infection. It follows, therefore, that paying attention to the early signals of infection in the urinary tract can frequently make the difference between becoming seriously ill and being able to avoid hospitalization and loss of time from daily activities.

Fever is an early warning of infection, both before and after an injury to the spinal cord. For most people without spinal cord injury, body temperature is about 98.6. However, "normal" temperature for a person with spinal cord injury, may be considerably lower; for that person, a temperature elevation to the range of 98 may be definitely *abnormal* and a sign of infection. You must know what is normal for you and recognize that it is significant when your temperature is no longer within its normal range. Other warnings of urinary tract infection are retention of urine in the bladder and a decrease in output, and an increase in spasticity in abdominal muscles and legs. In short, any unusual occurrence connected with the urinary system is a reason to seek help as quickly as possible. Of course, warnings of trouble, such as blood in the urine or thick, cloudy foul smelling urine with a lot of sediment apply equally to injured and uninjured persons.

COMMON URINARY PROBLEMS

People with spinal cord injuries are at increased risk for many problems related to urinary function. The most common problem is *urinary tract infection.* Symptoms of urinary tract infection (UTI) include elevated temperature, chills, a lack of energy, and changes in the odor and appearance of your urine. If you suspect that you have a urinary tract infection, contact your physician immediately so that you can begin taking medication to combat the infection before it becomes serious.

Another serious problem for some people is that of kidney stones, or *renal calculi.* If you have a tendency toward recurring kidney stones, medication can be used as a preventive measure to prevent additional episodes. However, existing stones must be removed through a small incision in the abdomen (*percutaneous nephrostomy*), general surgery, or by a new procedure called *extracorporeal shock wave lithotripsy* (ESWL), in which the person is placed in a large tub of water and shock waves are emitted to disintegrate the stones noninvasively. This procedure requires less hospitalization and less recovery time than traditional surgery.

Reflux occurs when urine backs up from the bladder into the kidney either because the bladder is not being emptied properly or because of infection or malfunctioning muscles in the urinary structure. Reflux can cause serious damage to the kidneys, and must be dealt with by a physician.

SUMMARY

The importance of adequate prevention and treatment of urinary tract infection and resulting complications such as kidney stone development cannot be overemphasized. You may not see the effects of what you are doing for 10 to 15 years. Like many parts of the body, a lot of room for error exists. However, repeated infections and kidney stone formation can lead to kidney failure, which may require removal of a damaged kidney or the need for dialysis. While dialysis can prolong life by keeping the body free of wastes, patients must spend long periods hooked up to the machine that "washes" the blood, just as the kidneys used to do. It requires about 8 hours of dialysis several times a week to maintain adequate cleansing.

Impending kidney failure is detected by laboratory blood tests or by x-rays, both of which must be conducted by experts in hospitals. But there are early warning signals which you can identify for yourself. It is important that you learn about these and be alert for them so that medical intervention can be provided *before* you reach the stage of kidney failure. One of the major purposes of a medical checkup is to monitor blood and do x-rays of various sorts to determine how well your kidneys are functioning. But even these signals come late, although not quite as late as the feelings of weakness and nausea, which come even later. The first line of defense for your kidneys is to keep your bladder washed out, and monitor changes in your urine. Finally, make sure to get help when you think you need it.

SUGGESTED READINGS

Jeter, K., ed.: *The HIP Report* (quarterly). Help for Incontinent People, P.O. Box 544, Union, SC 29739.

Jeter, K. (ed.) (Winter 1985—2nd ed.): *Resource Guide of Continence Aids and Services*. Help for Incontinent People, P.O. Box 544, Union, SC 29739.

CHAPTER 9

Managing Your Bowels

Mark N. Ozer with M. Elizabeth Bayless

HOW THE SYSTEM WORKS

After food is broken down into material that can be absorbed by the body in the stomach and small intestine, the large intestine is responsible for transforming the relatively liquid waste into feces, which is then excreted. Development of firm wastes is important. If wastes remain in the liquid form in which they enter the ascending portion of the large bowel, a great deal of water will be lost from the body. Very loose bowel movements, or diarrhea, can lead to dehydration. For many persons with spinal cord injury, loose bowel movements also are the cause of breakdown of their skin on buttocks.

AMOUNT OF FLUID

Although wastes must be solid to avoid leakage, they must not be so firm and with so much water removed that the feces are small and hard. The term "constipation" means different things to different people. Some people consider themselves to be constipated if they move their bowels less frequently than some arbitrary standard, such as every day. What is meant here is the consistency of the feces rather than the frequency of bowel movements. A person is considered to be constipated if the feces have stayed in the bowels a long time and appear hard.

If your bowels do not move regularly and completely, there is an increased likelihood of leakage, because relatively loose and watery wastes back up behind the blockage, and leakage occurs. The most common cause of diarrhea in persons with spinal cord injury is a blockage called a "fecal impaction," that is, the stool becomes so hard that it cannot move through the rectum.

To prevent impaction and resultant diarrhea and to avoid leakage at other times, stools should be soft but well-formed. Foods that are helpful in accomplishing this goal are those that provide "bulk," such as bran and whole wheat (see Table 9.2 for the fiber content of foods). Many laxatives work the same way, by holding water in the intestine. Water plus the bulk of fiber in your diet need to work together. One needs to have enough fluid in the diet in order for the fiber in the diet or laxatives to do their job.

MUSCLE ACTION

The walls of the large intestine contain muscles that contract and move the feces down the intestines to the storage area (rectum), and when defecation is to occur these muscles in the rectal wall help empty the bowel completely (Fig. 9.1).

The muscles in the intestinal wall are controlled by the nervous system. When the spinal cord is injured there is a cutoff of the usual control by the brain to the nerves going to the spinal cord and from there to the walls of the intestine. During spinal shock the intestine stops working (*paralytic ileus*). The intestine no longer contracts, and the sign of return of function is the return of "bowel sounds," ordinarily heard with a stethoscope.

Contraction of the intestine can be affected by medications. During spinal shock, medications such as *prostigmine* are nec-

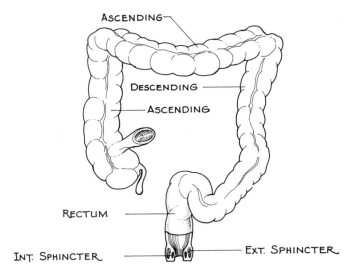

FIG. 9.1. The large intestine and rectum.

essary to stimulate the muscles and help prevent the intestine from becoming distended. When taking medication it is important to know whether it will change the action of the intestine. Medications used to paralyze the bladder, such as Pro-Banthine, may affect the bowels in the same way and it is important to prevent problems with one's bowels if such medications are otherwise necessary.

Fortunately, you will be able to regain the ability of the muscles in the intestinal wall to move the stools down to the storage area. It generally helps to regain such function if you are turned regularly, exercise as much as possible, and massage your abdomen. The return of the bowel to its previous action, now independent of the upper levels of the nervous system, includes the important reflex associated with the ingestion of food.

Many people have noted that the stool comes down to the colon soon after a meal. This "gastrocolic reflex" is not clearly understood in terms of whether it works by the nervous system connections or by blood-carried hormones. Studies show that this reflex is available for persons with spinal cord injury, regardless of the level of injury. This association with the ingestion of food can therefore be used to increase the likelihood of controlling the timing of the bowel program just as it might have done for the person before injury to the spinal cord.

The important actions of the colon are the absorption of fluids, the movement of the increasingly formed stool through the intestines to the colon, and the storage of stool in the colon before defecation, and all these functions are either retained or quickly reestablished in the person with a spinal cord injury. Knowing how the body absorbs fluids and moves the stool down to the storage area are two aspects that can provide you with several important means of controlling what has been affected right after injury.

The muscles in the wall of the rectum need to contract to help expel the feces and open up the anus which is controlled by a muscle called the anal sphincter. This is usually a double muscle, the internal and external sphincter. When SCI occurs, it usually is this coordinated action of the rectum and the sphincter that is most affected; the smooth operation between them has been lost as well as the sensation of "fullness."

The effects of damage to the spinal cord generally vary depending on the location and severity of the injury. Emptying the bowels is coordinated at the levels of S2 to S4 (Figure 9.2), at the very end of the spinal cord. Injury or damage at this level may enable the eventual development of what has been called *automatic* defecation. The procedures to be followed by the person with damage at this level to regain control over the bowels will be different from those persons with damage to the spinal cord above S2.

Damage above S2 is much more common, and eventually enables the person to develop what is called *reflex* defecation, a term meaning that coordination of the actions of the rectum and the sphincter remains available. However, the connection

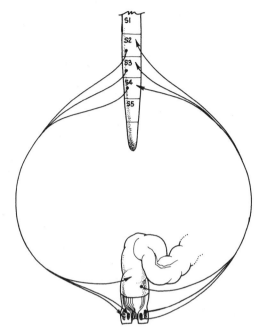

FIG. 9.2. Bowel function is controlled at the sacral level of the spinal cord.

between this coordinating center, called the "defecation center," and the brain has been severed.

REFLEX DEFECATION

Before injury, sensations of "fullness" or "touch" or "pain" come from the rectum, signaling a need to defecate. When the spinal cord is injured, that signal no longer reaches consciousness. The person is not aware of the need to defecate or of fullness, nor of the presence of stool in the rectum, nor even of defecation.

When the spinal cord is injured above the level of the defecation center S2, the external sphincter stays closed all the time. Ways must be devised to open it in coordination with the contraction of the rectal portion of the bowel, and do so at the chosen time and place.

One technique to achieve this is to bear down and to increase pressure within the abdominal cavity. Those with relatively low levels of injury (below T5) and therefore with fairly intact abdominal wall muscles can use those muscles to bear down. In the absence of good abdominal muscles, manual pressure can be used to achieve similar results. The increase in intraabdominal pressure, if maintained, causes the external sphincter to open and the rectal wall to contract, and it brings about a reflex evacuation of the bowels.

Filling the rectum itself will eventually cause contraction of the rectal wall and opening up of the external sphincter. The task in general is to have the stool in the storage area ready to be emptied from this lower tract.

One way to encourage the body to release the stool is to apply digital stimulation. When a finger is inserted into the anus, the external sphincter contracts and then relaxes in a person with injury to the spinal cord, as it did for that same person before injury. With injury, relaxation after the initial contraction is more prompt and lasts longer after stretching.

A bowel care program for those with injury to the spinal cord above S2, therefore, includes careful attention to diet, and possibly the use of laxatives taken by mouth serve to bring about a sufficiently bulky stool. The use of massage and exercise and avoidance of medications that slow down the bowel help bring about movement of the feces through the intestine to the storage area. Recognition of the connection between intake of food and movement of the bowel muscles helps with the timing of the bowel program. After eating, bowel contents are transferred to the storage area of the colon.

A local, stimulant-type laxative can be used at first to increase the likelihood of contraction. Eventually a glycerin suppository is all that will be needed to aid evacuation. Thus, the goal of regular, prompt, and complete evacuation of the bowels at a chosen time and place can be met for those persons with spinal cord involvement above the level of the defecation center. The results are the same as before injury, but the methods require a greater awareness of the way the system works.

BOWEL MANAGEMENT IN SACRAL INJURIES

It is important to note here that failure to empty your bowels regularly can lead to a serious health problem called *autonomic dysreflexia* (see Chapter 11), particularly for people with higher level injuries. Consequently, regular and complete evacuation of bowels is an even more important health consideration for people with spinal cord injuries than it was before.

Now let us turn to the much less common situation, when the level of injury to the spinal cord is in the region of the sacral cord, the level of the defecation center. After injury at this level, a person can still regain control over evacuation of the bowels so that movements occur at a chosen time and place. The means are somewhat different from those described above because several of the muscles are acting less strongly and the reflex effects of digital stimulation are unavailable. Defecation still requires the interplay of an increase in intra-abdominal pressure, opening of the sphincter holding the anus closed, and contraction of the wall of the rectum propelling the fecal contents.

Contraction of the rectal wall can still occur but does not do so as strongly as with injuries at the higher levels of the spinal cord. Similarly, the muscle acting to provide closure of the anus is slower and less effective than that available with higher injuries. The only muscle that continues to act in injuries in the region of the sacral cord is the internal sphincter, whereas in the higher level of injury both this and another, more active external sphincter are present.

Pressure buildup in this level of injury is too low to depend on the rectal wall to do the job, and at times it becomes necessary to remove the feces with a gloved finger as well as use the intraabdominal pressure. Because there is less closure available with the sphincters, it becomes even more important to use techniques to prevent leakage and constipation by completely emptying the colon after the stool of the proper consistency has been removed. It becomes even more important to use the storage capability of the bowel because the last line of defense against fecal incontinence has been lost.

It is also important to prevent excessive distention of the rectum early in the course of your injury and to prevent distension in general so that whatever action the rectal wall can take in contraction is not lost. Avoid foods and drugs that may cause diarrhea because the opportunity for fecal incontinency is more likely. Knowing how to carry out digital evacuation so that it does not cause injury to the rectum and anus with consequent infection and the possibility of hemorrhoids is also critical.

MANAGING YOUR BOWEL PROGRAM

In regaining control over your bowels, you will need to define your own concerns. The results you want may be somewhat different from those of another person. Your priorities will be based on your own particular lifestyle. Please note that the use of enemas is not necessary to manage one's bowels regardless of the level of injury. What are your priorities and your goals? Is the goal to be the prevention of accidents at all costs? Is your goal to be able to take a relatively short defecation time but to do so more frequently?

One person may be particularly concerned about having accidents in public and the embarrassment that it can cause. No one wants to have an accident at any time. Another concern of people with spinal cord injury is being able to complete a bowel control program within a reasonable length of time; they don't want it to interfere with their ability to schedule other things on the same day, such as work or recreation. Most people find that 30 minutes every other day is enough time to complete the process.

In addition to the dual goals of avoiding accidents and not taking too much time, people with spinal cord injury need to be able to plan their bowel care. One way to learn what works for you is to keep a diary for several weeks. By keeping a daily record of your activities, you will quickly learn the best times, best amounts, and best kinds of food to encourage bowel control. Medications such as laxatives and stool softeners should not be necessary at all times nor for everyone. They are available as they were before your injury, and as then you should keep their use under your control. Learn how your system reacts to these medications, and *you* decide whether to use them. In general a given laxative will work more slowly, overnight for example, if one uses less and will work in a few hours with larger doses. The techniques, usually unconscious, which may have worked for you before your injury are no longer sufficient. At least at the start you need to be more aware of the techniques that are available for you to regain control. Once you know what you are doing, you can once again do what you want.

As with urinary system management and every other routine bodily function, management of the bowels should not control one's life or limit participation in other activities. The key to relegating bowel movements to a routine role in life is knowledge about the system itself and use of that knowledge to make decisions about your own personal approach to bowel care.

FIBER IN YOUR DIET[a]

Fiber is the part of plants which is not broken down by chemical action in the digestive system. Fiber is sometimes referred to as bulk or roughage, and is important in bowel regulation and control. Fiber increases the bulk and softens the consistency of your stool by holding water in the stool. Bulky, softer stools are easier to pass through the intestinal

---

[a] This section was written by M. Elizabeth Bayless.

TABLE 9.1. *Sample high-fiber menu*[a]

	Food	Amount	Fiber
Breakfast	Fresh orange	1 Medium	2.8
	Scrambled egg	One	0.0
	All bran	⅔ Cup	17.0
	Whole wheat toast	2 Slices	4.2
	Margarine	2 Teaspoons	—
	Marmalade	1 Tablespoon	Trace
	Milk	1 Cup	0.0
	Coffee		0.0
			24.0
Lunch	Sliced turkey	2 Ounces	0.0
	Whole wheat bread	2 Slices	4.2
	Sliced tomato	2 Slices (½ small)	0.4
	Salad: lettuce	½ Cup	1.0
	Cucumber	¼ Medium	—
	Green peppers	¼ Large	—
	French dressing	2 Tablespoons	—
	Fresh apple	1 Medium	2.8
	Iced tea		—
			8.4
Supper	Broiled haddock	4 Ounces	—
	Baked potato with skin	1 Medium	2.5
	Broccoli	⅔ Cup	4.1
	Raw carrot sticks	½ Cup	1.5
	Bran muffin	1 Medium	3.5
	Margarine	1 Teaspoon	—
	Milk	1 Cup	—
	Fresh pear	1 Medium	4.1
			15.7

[a] Total fiber for the day: 48.1 grams.

tract. Easily passed stools make your bowel care routine simple.

The average American diet contains about 20 grams of dietary fiber. You will need to increase the fiber in your diet to much more. You can aim for about 40 grams each day as about right, but every person differs (Tables 9.1 and 9.2).

Select whole grain breads and cereals, fresh fruits, and raw

TABLE 9.2. *Fiber chart*

Fiber may be measured as either crude fiber or dietary fiber. This chart lists values for dietary fiber of some common foods. Cup = 8-ounce measure.

Food	Amount	Grams of dietary fiber
Bread and cereals		
All Bran	⅔ Cup	17.0
Bran Buds	⅔ Cup	15.8
Branflakes	¾ Cup	4.0
Cornflakes	1 Cup	0.5
Grape Nuts	½ Cup	2.8
Oatmeal	¾ Cup	1.6
Puffed wheat	1 Cup	0.5
Rice Krispies	1 Cup	0.1
Shredded wheat	1 Biscuit	2.2
Special K	⅔ Cup	0.1
Whole wheat bread	1 Slice	2.1
White bread	1 Slice	0.7
Bran muffin	1 Medium	3.5
Fruits		
Apple, raw with skin	1 Medium	2.8
Applesauce	½ Cup	1.4
Apricots, raw	3 Medium	1.4
Apricots, canned	6 Halves	.8
Banana, raw	1 Medium	1.6
Blackberries, raw	½ Cup	3.3
Cantaloupe, raw	1 Cup	0.5
Grapefruit, raw	½	0.5
Orange	1 Medium	2.8
Peach, raw	1 Medium	0.5
Peach, canned	½ Cup	0.5
Pear, raw	1 Medium	4.1
Pear, canned	½ Cup	1.2
Pineapple, canned	½ Cup	.9
Prunes, dried	4	5.4
Strawberries, raw	1 Cup	2.8
Vegetables		
Asparagus	½ Cup	1.5
Avocado, raw	½ Medium	2.3
Beans, green	½ Cup	2.0
Broccoli, cooked	⅔ Cup	4.1
Brussel sprouts, cooked	6–8 Medium	2.9

TABLE 9.2.   *Fiber chart* (contd.)

Food	Amount	Grams of dietary fiber
Vegetables (*contd.*)		
Cabbage, raw	½ Cup	1.7
Carrots, raw	1 Large	2.9
Carrots, cooked	⅔ Cup	3.1
Cauliflower, raw	½ Cup	1.0
Cauliflower, cooked	½ Cup	1.1
Celery, raw	2 Stalks	1.8
Corn on cob	4-Inch ear	4.7
Cucumbers	1 Medium	0.4
Lettuce	3½ Ounces	1.5
Mushrooms	10 Small	2.5
Peas, green, canned	⅔ Cup	6.3
Peppers, green	¼ Large	.2
Potato, baked	1 Medium	2.5
Potatoes, mashed	½ Cup	.9
Spinach, cooked	½ Cup	6.3
Tomato, raw	1 Small	1.5
Tomato, canned	⅖ Cup	0.9
Other		
Graham Crackers	4 Squares	0.8
Ryekrisp	2 Triple crackers	1.6
Wheat Snacks	15	1.1

or crisp tender vegetables. Begin your high-fiber diet by adding one to two high-fiber foods to your usual diet. If after 3 to 4 days, your stools are still hard or you have diarrhea with impacted stool, increase to three high-fiber foods. Continue to add high-fiber foods every 3 to 4 days until your stools become soft and bulky.

Fluid is very important. Since fiber traps water in your stools to form a gel-like bulk, you must drink plenty of fluid. Drink at least eight 8-ounce glasses of water, juice, or other liquid daily. (If your routine bowel care is in the morning, start the day with a cup of hot coffee or tea or a glass of warm water. This encourages the normal motions of the bowel and should make passage of your stool easier.)

SUGGESTED READING

Cheever, R. C., and Elmer, C. D. (eds.): *Bowel Management Programs— A Manual of Ideas and Techniques*. Accent Special Publications, Accent on Living, Inc., P.O. Box 700, Bloomington, IL 61701.

CHAPTER 10

Skin Care

Mark N. Ozer

Many people with spinal cord injury have difficulties with their skin. Skin problems can limit your ability to function on the job or to care for yourself. Even relatively minor skin problems can require an average of 4 months of hospitalization. More severe problems, such as infections that have invaded the bone, may need surgery and a long hospital stay.

Improved nursing techniques and the availability of antibiotics have reduced life-threatening skin problems dramatically, but infections from skin breakdown can still involve the bone and kidneys. Once the infection is underway it may be very resistant to antibiotics and other drugs.

HOW THE SYSTEM WORKS

The skin protects the body from the loss of fluids and serves as a barrier to infection and injury to the deeper structures. The skin is an organ, which has several layers serving different functions (Fig. 10.1). The outermost layer, called the *epidermis*, is the one that you touch and see, and it provides the protection you want to maintain. The epidermal layer is continually producing cells that provide protection on the surface as the older cells wear out. The older cells are in direct contact with the environment and are continually being rubbed off and replaced. The cells in the epidermis produce cells throughout life, one of only a few places where this occurs.

124

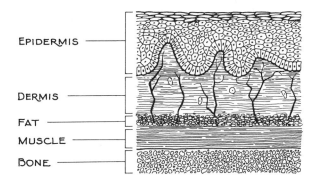

FIG. 10.1. Cross sections of human skin and bone tissue.

The next layer, called the *dermis*, contains the blood vessels that provide nourishment to the crucial cellular layer over them. If an injury to the skin involves this dermal layer, a scar will form when healing occurs. The degree of scarring depends somewhat on the degree to which the blood vessels have been destroyed.

Below the dermis is the fat that provides a cushion between the outside epidermal layer and the underlying muscles and bone. If an injury to the skin goes into these deeper structures of muscle and bone, healing is more difficult because the protection the outside layers need to cushion the pressure of the bone is not available. It therefore becomes necessary to replace this lost muscle by transplant or graft from an adjacent area.

As far as we know, the skin of a person with an injury to the spinal cord functions the same as it did before injury, with the exception of the first few days after injury when the blood vessels feeding the skin are more subject to compression. The health of any part of the body depends on the cells getting enough oxygen and nutrients, and on adequate removal of waste products—the job of the blood supply.

The blood supply system pumps blood from the heart through the large vessels and then through smaller arteries to

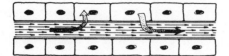

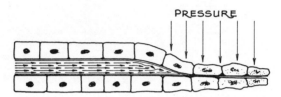

FIG. 10.2. Pressure can inhibit flow of blood to skin cells and lead to cell death.

the very smallest vessels, called capillaries, which carry blood directly to the cells (Fig. 10.2). Blood flowing through the capillaries brings the red blood cells carrying oxygen and nutrients into direct contact with the cells and also carries away the waste products. It is this layer of blood vessels in the dermal layer of the skin—the capillary bed—that you can see change when the blood supply is affected.

Any increase in blood flow causes a flushing of the skin, similar to blushing. The opposite is when your skin looks pale or even white when any pressure reduces the blood flowing through the capillary bed. Very little pressure is required to block off this capillary bed, causing the waste products to build up and the cell to die.

Fortunately, tissues such as skin do not die even at very high pressures if pressure is relieved often enough. If a sufficient rest period is given to the tissues between pressure applications, the blood flowing back through the capillary bed can bring the nutrients needed and flush out the waste products. Death of tissue can generally be avoided even with only partial relief for short periods. However, very high pressures such as those produced by sitting on a hard surface are obviously dangerous. There are no guarantees that the blood flowing back will do so soon enough.

After the blood flows through the capillaries and has dropped off the nutrients and picked up the waste products, it flows through slightly larger vessels, called venules, and then through lymphatic channels and the larger veins back to the heart. When a person slides along the sheet in bed rather than being lifted, the surface of the skin slides along but the part further away does not. This separation action, called "shearing," tears the connection between the capillary bed and the larger vessels both as they bring nutrients and take away waste products. Large areas of skin can be undermined in this way.

After a partial or short-term blockage of the capillary bed or the veins draining back to the heart, blood flow will increase to try to compensate, a condition called reactive *hyperemia*; the size of the capillary bed increases to carry the increased load, resulting in a local blush or redness. If the redness disappears when you press on the area, the blood is still within the capillary walls, a good sign that with relief from further pressure the skin tissue will live. If the blockage has been complete and lengthy, you will see some redness that does not go away easily or at all when you press on it, and some swelling may be evident. What has happened is that red blood cells and fluid, which had been contained within the walls of the capillaries, have escaped into the tissues surrounding these very thin-walled vessels. The size of the sore and its depth will vary with the degree of swelling and how the pressure affects the death of further tissue. There is still a chance, albeit a slim one, that if no further pressure is exerted the tissue will recover. That is why it is absolutely essential to check your skin as often as possible when you get into bed after sitting or after lying in bed all night, so that you can respond immediately to the first signs of trouble.

You must know, too, where to look first when checking your skin. Pressure is greater when applied to a small area

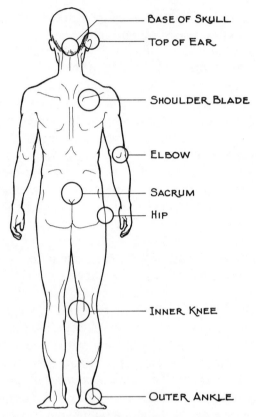

FIG. 10.3. Bony prominences are most susceptible to tissue damage.

than when it is spread over a large one. Compare the pain you feel when pressing all your weight on the palm of your hand and when putting all your weight on the knuckle of one finger. The pain, and the pressure which causes such pain, is greatest over what are called pressure points. These are usually points where your bones are more prominent and closer to the surface of your body (Fig. 10.3). When lying on your back, the base of your spine is one such area. When sitting in a chair the ischial (lower hip) bones stick out and bear more than their share of pressure. When lying on your side the bones of the upper thigh protrude, making this an area subject to early skin breakdown. Figure 10.3 shows a number of areas where pressure is likely to concentrate. These are the areas you should check most often. Other important areas for surveillance are those that might rub against the sheets, such as the heels and buttocks. Persons with specific patterns of contracture or spasticity will have their pressure points at places somewhat different from the usual.

So far we have described the effects of pressure on the outside layer of skin and the blood vessels directly beneath this outside layer. Even deeper is the layer of fat and muscle that provides the cushion between the outside skin and the bone. These tissues are even more vulnerable to a blockage of blood supply. If pressure is applied at the point of the bone as you lie or sit on it, the effects of that pressure increase when the tissue is closer to the bone. The deeper tissues of fat and muscle may die over a wide area, whereas on the surface of the skin the area that dies is much smaller. This explains why a relatively small area of breakdown on the skin may fail to indicate the real extent of the tissue death beneath.

A "knot" in the skin or deeper down close to the bone is an early sign of breakdown even if the skin looks and feels normal. To recognize the early signs of breakdown, it is necessary to feel as well as look when you check your skin.

Any skin breakdown must be taken seriously, regardless of its apparently minor extent on the surface, and immediate steps must be taken to relieve the pressure. Pressure points also relate to what can happen over time when constant pressure leads to a thickening and hardness in what is called the *bursa* of the bone. The bursa, a padlike sac is normally found over the *ischial tuberosities* and the *trochanter*, the bony areas around the hip region. With the thickening and possible swelling of this tissue, the degree of prominence of the bone in that area may increase even further. Thus, when you lie or sit, the degree to which pressure is localized to that area increases.

Breakdown in these areas in which a bursa has formed will heal only to break down again almost immediately when any pressure is applied. Failure to heal when pressure relief has been used in either of these problems is an important reason to seek help.

The first goal for any person with spinal cord injury is to prevent skin breakdown. If injury to the skin does occur, the next goal is to know immediately that it has occurred and to deal with it to prevent deep layers of skin and larger areas becoming involved. The third goal is to know when to seek medical care and/or surgery as part of the treatment.

An ulcer in the skin is the same as the death of some skin. The dead skin (and then the tissue beneath it) becomes infected and then more and more skin dies. The progress of skin ulceration is a vicious cycle. Sometimes, it begins with a little injury to a very small area, caused by something as innocuous as a crumb in the bed or a wrinkled sheet. Once the skin has been broken, it is important to prevent further damage.

PREVENTION

The things that can injure the skin are the same for people with spinal injuries as those for any other person. Too much heat will burn; too much cold will cause frostbite; cuts and bruises cause pain and require time to heal; sitting on hard or sharp objects is no good for anyone anytime; and lying in a pool of urine or feces never did anyone's skin any good. The difference is that if you have an injury to the spinal cord, you won't necessarily know when the bath water is too hot or a sharp object is pressing against your leg, because the sensations of touch and pain and temperature are frequently disconnected from the rest of the body. To overcome this disadvantage, you must develop and expand the use of other senses such as vision, and use the feelings of touch still intact. For most people with spinal cord injuries, the senses of touch and pressure are no longer fully intact. Nonetheless, other signals exist and may replace those that you had before your injury. Many say that a sense of "burning" is their signal that they have been sitting too long in one position. It is important to react to that signal early and not wait for the burning feeling to spread. The goal is to relieve pressure often enough to prevent the burning from ever appearing. Others have noted that an increase in the usual level of their spasticity is a signal to move.

Although signals are frequently available, the problem is to attend to them and consciously act on something that did not ordinarily reach the level of awareness before injury. You may find it useful to use a timing device to remind you to shift weight in the absence of any consistent signal from your body. Regardless of the technique used, the goal is the same—to avoid injury to the skin by thinking and acting in ways that will take the place of the almost automatic shifting that people do ordinarily. Once the technique of attending to a predetermined signal and responding to it by shifting has been established, many people find it semiautomatic and can later frequently do without external reminders.

EARLY IDENTIFICATION

In the event that preventive measures fail and skin becomes injured in some way, effort must be made to avoid involvement of the deeper layers of the skin and to heal the area that has been damaged. Whether the cause of the difficulty is a burn or pressure, the effects are the same. Skin responds to injury by first becoming red or dusky. This is true for persons with light or dark skin. Other early signs, but generally after the appearance of the redness, include roughness, often with an early break even before any visual evidence of an abrasion occurs. A pimple or blister is another early sign, just as it was evidence that something was wrong with your skin before injury to your spinal cord. For some, a "knot" deep near the bone comes even before evidence appears on the skin. It is important to look for these signs regularly, such as right after getting into bed and each time after sitting, and to know the areas where your bones are prominent and the skin more vulnerable.

The earlier you become aware of a skin problem and take defensive action, the more likely you are to prevent further difficulty. The first and most important treatment when any of these signs appear is relief of the pressure. Anything else is secondary.

In addition to being aware of the need to be constantly alert for skin eruptions, it is important to understand what you are looking for, where to look, how to inspect your skin (using a hand mirror, as necessary), and knowing what to do at the first sign of trouble.

The length of time it is safe to sit or to otherwise apply pressure to the skin without relief is the same for all people. Very few people remain in one position for longer than 10 or 15 minutes without shifting weight, and move even more often. The difference is that after injury you must make a conscious effort to move regularly because it will no longer be a reflex action.

WHEN TO GET HELP

The general principle for treatment of any ulcer is to keep it clean to avoid infection and to relieve the affected areas of any further pressure. It also is important to seek medical attention if it appears unlikely that the sore will heal itself. The signals for getting medical attention are the same as with any wound, e.g., pus or other evidence of infection, including chills or fever.

Depending upon the size, location, and severity of your sore, one or more treatment approaches may be used to heal the infected area. If a small ulcer does not heal, it is possible that a "sinus tract" has developed, which occurs because a connection into a deeper abscess exists. It may close over when you relieve the pressure but then break down again quickly with any sitting. It may need to be opened up and drained, which can be done easily in a hospital.

Some infections will need to be *debrided*, which involves scraping dead tissue from the infected area to remove bacteria and prevent further growth. The wound then will need to be kept clean and treated with medication to prevent infection.

Some wounds will require surgery. Generally, the deeper and wider the wound, the more likely it is that surgery will be necessary. This often involves replacing dead tissue from the infected area with healthy tissue from another part of the body.

The kinds of medications that are used to clean wounds, heal infections, and clear out dead tissue that can lead to future infection vary from person to person. If you have an episode of skin breakdown that requires medical attention, it would be helpful to you in the future to know what medications are used and why, so that you can understand the goals of your treatment. In addition, the general approach to healing any wound that you have had in the past still applies.

One additional factor that will influence how much dead tissue can be restored is the food you eat. Food—or more accurately, the right food—provides your body with the nutrients it needs to restore health to the affected area. It has been estimated that the amount of protein needed in the diet may be as high as 200 grams a day compared with the usual 50 grams for an adult without a spinal cord injury. Certain vitamins, such as A and C, may also be useful for wound healing.

Anything that decreases the amount of oxygen being carried to the tissues inhibits healing. Smoking is detrimental because nicotine in tobacco restricts the blood vessels carrying oxygen to the wound. This becomes particularly important when the wound is in an area such as the skin overlying the bony prominence of the ankle, which is a long way from the heart and has a relatively poor blood supply under the best conditions.

Also, breathing smoke that contains carbon monoxide from the incomplete burning of the cigarette can reduce the amount of oxygen available at the sites where it is needed. Any swelling or edema of the tissues also restricts the flow of oxygen from the capillaries to the damaged tissues, so elevation of the legs is an important part of the treatment of pressure ulcers on the feet.

The signals that people use to warn themselves about excess pressure to the skin vary, as does the frequency with which each individual needs to relieve pressure. Some people have tender skin; others, less so. The goal remains the same—to prevent any injury to your skin—and the ways you accomplish this will depend on your own personality and lifestyle. Skin breakdown is not inevitable if you have an injury to the spinal cord. If that were true, people with the most severe injuries would have the most trouble, and they don't. It really depends on how you use the senses that remain and how well you take charge of yourself.

SUGGESTED READINGS

National Symposium on the Care, Treatment and Prevention of Decubitus Ulcers (1984 Conference Proceedings). Available from Paralyzed Veterans of America, 801 Eighteenth St., N.W., Washington, DC 20006.

A Workshop on the Effects of Pressure on Human Tissue (1977). Rehabilitation Services Administration, Washington, DC 20201.

Zacharkow, D.: *Wheelchair Posture and Pressure Sores.* Charles C Thomas, Publisher, 2600 South First St., Springfield, IL 62717.

CHAPTER 11

Chronic Pain, Spasticity, and Autonomic Dysreflexia

Mark N. Ozer, Catherine W. Britell, and Lynn Phillips

The most obvious problems associated with spinal cord injury are those that relate to functions that have been lost or changed as a result of the injury, such as muscle strength and sensation. Several spinal cord injury–related problems, however, have no obvious preinjury counterpart, and thus are a bit more difficult to understand. These include (1) chronic pain below the level of the injury, (2) spasticity or uncontrollable movement below the level of injury, and (3) autonomic dysreflexia, which is a malfunction of the body's normal regulating mechanisms for blood pressure and temperature. All these problems are directly related to the disconnection that occurs in the spinal cord after an injury, and all can have disruptive influence on your life if you do not understand and treat them appropriately.

CHRONIC PAIN AND SPASTICITY

What Happens After Injury?

The central nervous system is very complex and functions through balancing and sorting messages that come from different regions of the brain and peripheral nervous system. As a result of these complex interactions, we are able to sort out the most important information coming from sensors in our skin and throughout many of our internal organs. Without any conscious thought, we normally receive vast quantities of information, sort through all this complex information, select those messages which are most important to our needs and act on them.

These "reflex" actions allow us to carry out many complex activities, virtually without thinking, reserving conscious thought for specialized activities that require our most sophisticated decision-making abilities. Much reflex activity is actually carried out in the lower reaches of the spinal cord, but is regulated by information sent down from the brain. Two of the most important purposes of this complex process of regulation are (1) filtering the vast amount of sensory information about touch, pain, and limb position that comes into the spinal cord and sorting out that which is most important and (2) defining control of limb and trunk muscles, which allows just the right amount of movement in response to a stimulus. This unconscious spinal cord processing allows us to direct our conscious attention only to major tasks, such as deciding which *kind* of movement to make or how to deal with the fact that we have cut a finger, for example.

In spinal cord injury, there is an interruption in the delicate interplay between sensation, reflex, and controlled movement, which prevents both transmission of sensations to the brain where conscious feeling actually takes place and transmission of commands about movement to the spinal reflex centers (Fig. 11.1). However, this interruption does not prevent continuing receipt and processing of sensory information below the site of damage. It merely prevents the passage of such information to and from the centers of consciousness higher in the brain.

Without normal interplay of information, both the reflex centers in the spinal cord and the information-processing centers in the brain eventually begin to malfunction in subtle but often annoying and debilitating ways. These malfunctions are

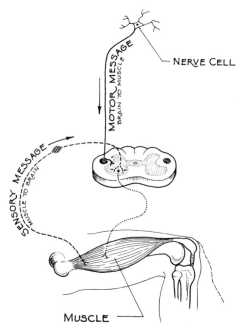

FIG. 11.1. Normal transmission of messages between muscles and brain. Spinal cord injury interrupts these pathways.

perceived as (1) inappropriate sensations of "pain" without obvious sources of tissue damage that could be alleviated and (2) inappropriate muscle contractions, or spasticity.

These symptoms do not appear immediately after a spinal cord injury; they develop over time as the nervous system gradually adapts to the lack of communication between its parts. The detailed neuromechanisms responsible for controlling movement and the perception of pain are still poorly understood, even by scientists.

In order to react appropriately to the new sensations one experiences after a spinal cord injury and to control movements as effectively as possible under these new circumstances, it is important for the spinal cord–injured person to understand as much as possible about how his or her particular body reacts to various stimuli.

Understanding Chronic Pain

The character of chronic pain is quite different from that sort of pain that comes from a cut or some other acute injury. Acute pain is a signal of injury to the body and serves an obvious biological need; chronic pain serves no such useful purpose.

Various kinds of pain may occur in a person with a spinal cord injury. One kind, *mechanical pain*, is usually sharp, comes from a specific and usually small area, and is often aggravated by bending, twisting, lifting, or jarring. It is seldom constant. It can come from bones, ligaments, tendons, joints, or nerve roots at the site of the injury. This type of pain may indicate an unstable fracture site, pinched nerve, or arthritis of the spine and should receive a careful medical evaluation. Another kind of pain that is sometimes seen is that which is not localized to the site of the injury but may be due to arthritis or other inflammation of joints and tendons or to contractures (muscles that tighten up and are difficult to relax). These can be treated directly and will often respond to a physical therapy regimen. A type of abnormal sensation specific to those with spinal cord injury, which is sometimes perceived as painful, is called *spinal cord disasthesia*, or *phantom sensation*. Its cause is not precisely known. Ninety-five percent of people who have had a spinal cord injury feel some tingling, burning, or dull aches in their back, legs, or feet at some time. This usually becomes of less and less concern as time goes on. However, 10 to 15 percent of people find this problem persistently bothersome and a few find it disabling.

This kind of pain can be affected by the weather, anxiety, depression, stress, smoking, coffee drinking, and many other nonspecific variables. Just like vision and hearing, pain is a sensory phenomenon, and just as some people see and hear more sharply than others, pain may be felt more sharply by some people than others.

Treatment of Chronic Pain

Because all brains and all spinal cord injuries are to some extent unique, the actual type of inappropriate sensation experienced by each individual can be varied. When sensations of pain continue over a long period of time, they can be a major burden. The first step in treatment is a careful medical evaluation to find and correct any specific problems. Then, often a combination of treatments is the best way to improve one's comfort level. These may include physical therapy and exercise, relaxation training, psychotherapy, medications, and dietary improvement. One should be very cautious about using pain medications, as they can often cause more problems then they solve. Although narcotics can sometimes make a person "feel better" initially, they are universally addicting, cause severe constipation, and usually have no effect on the pain itself, especially when used longer than 4 to 6 weeks. In addition, it has been found that many pain medications block the body's very potent natural pain-killing substances, and therefore often actually make chronic pain worse.

Transcutaneous electrical nerve stimulation (TENS), antidepressant medications, and antiseizure medications are often effectively used to block pain transmission in the nerves and spinal cord. Other substances, such as large doses of vitamins, industrial solvents (DMSO), marijuana or alcohol, which some people have tried for pain relief, can be dangerous and should be avoided.

In general, good stretching, avoidance of skin ulcers, good nutrition, and optimal bladder and bowel care are the first steps in treatment. When pain is causing significant suffering, psychological care, possibly including relaxation training, psychotherapy, focusing and imagery, and family therapy is often very helpful. The goal of this combined treatment is to achieve optimal physical, psychological, and social functioning.

Understanding Spasticity

During the first 4 to 6 weeks after spinal cord injury, the usual period of spinal shock, the area of the spinal cord below the level of injury responds by loss of all function. There are no reflexes during this time and the muscles innervated below the level of the injury are floppy or *flaccid*. As time passes, usually during the second month after injury, the spinal cord gradually regains independent reflex activity below the level of injury, whether or not there is also a return of voluntary muscle activity. The reflex activity is greater than what had been present before the injury, and this exaggeration of normal responses makes up what is called spasticity.

The reflex action of the spinal cord is divided into three parts. The first is the sensory phase, which is the input of information from the skin, muscles, or joints to the spinal cord. This input comes into the spinal cord just as it did before the injury; however, it does not reach the brain because of the interruption in the spinal cord, so the person remains unaware of the stimulus. However, it is important to remember that there has been no loss of the ability to have this input carried by the nerves from the skin, muscle, and joints into the spinal cord.

The second step of reflex action is the phase in which the information that comes in is organized and prioritized so that a response of the proper type and degree will result. The disconnection between the brain and spinal cord causes a severe problem at this point because signals from below the level of injury cannot get through to the brain and controlling signals from the brain cannot get through to the appropriate spinal cord level.

The third step of the reflex is the output, or *motor response*. This is relatively unaffected by the disconnection between the spinal cord and the brain. The nerves leading out of the spinal cord to the muscles are intact below the level of the injury. The muscles themselves are generally unaffected, except the wasting that occurs from lack of use.

Thus, while the muscle action continues to be possible after spinal cord injury, the coordination of the muscle response that comes from the brain and upper spinal cord no longer occurs. The end result is a highly exaggerated response to a stimulus, which is not a functional motion.

An example of this is the *flexor-reflex*, or withdrawal reflex. If the bottom or side of the foot is stimulated painfully, the foot draws away from the unpleasant sensation. This is brought about by flexion of the ankle, knee, and hip and is the characteristic flexor pattern that we see in many people after spinal cord injury. A flexor spasm may occur as a result of a number of stimuli—a burn, a pressure sore, bladder infections, or impacted bowels, to name just a few. Sometimes flexor spasms occur with what may seem to be insignificant stimuli, such as a light touch on the leg, or some other non-painful stimulus, and sometimes there appears to be no reason for the flexor spasm. Thus, we see spasticity as an *exaggerated*, or *inappropriate*, reaction to a stimulus below the level of the injury.

The Management of Spasticity

The three important concepts to keep in mind in dealing with spasticity are as follows: (1) Spasticity can be useful in telling you about a problem below the level of your injury. (2) Spasticity can be helpful to you in doing transfers and maintaining muscle bulk. (3) Spasticity should be treated only if it is getting in the way of your optimal lifestyle.

We all use pain sensations to warn us that something is wrong. Although you will have reduced sensation to such painful stimuli below the level of your spinal cord injury, you can use spasticity as a tool for knowing that something may be wrong, even though you may not immediately be aware of the source of the problem. By looking at spasms as a source of information about potential problems—bladder infection, the beginning of a pressure sore, shoes that are too tight, and so on—you will be using the signals of spasticity to monitor your body and your health.

Moderate spasticity has other benefits. It can be helpful in maintaining muscle bulk below the level of injury, and it is possible to use your spasms to assist in transferring or in standing. The most important thing is to learn how your body reacts in various situations and then use that information to achieve your goals.

If spasticity increases, the first thing to do is to look for the cause. It may be a bladder infection, a bowel impaction, tight shoes, the beginning of a pressure sore, or some other condition that would normally be painful to you. When you have made certain that all the possible sources of trouble have been treated or eliminated, then you will need to decide whether to treat your spasticity. Proper stretching is one of the most important ways to diminish nonuseful spasticity. Complete stretching of muscles at least daily or sometimes twice daily can make them less sensitive to the stimuli which cause spasticity. For many people with spinal cord injury, standing in a standing frame or standing or walking with braces have also been noted to decrease nonfunctional spasticity.

If a specific treatment for spasticity is used, the important objective is to interfere as little as possible with normal function. Three medications that are used to control spasticity are Baclofen, Diazepam, and Dantrolene. Baclofen seems to interfere the least with daily functioning, and its positive effect is variable. It acts within the spinal cord to dampen the overexcited response to stimuli entering the spinal cord. Another drug which acts in a different way in the brain and the spinal cord is Diazepam. This drug is quite effective in decreasing spasticity; however, it is also a very potent depressant and will tend to make one sleepy and less energetic, and it sometimes impairs judgment. In some instances, Diazepam and Baclofen are used together and are effective in managing severe spasticity. Dantrolene works at the level of the muscle response and causes a generalized weakening of all muscles. Therefore, this drug is usually most disruptive of normal movement and is usually reserved for those people who have a very high level injury and little or no functional movement and who need control of spasticity for wheelchair positioning and hygiene.

Another medication which is presently undergoing study for treatment of spasticity is Clonidine. This medication, when used in a number of spastic spinal cord–injured patients for control of blood pressure, was found to be associated with a decrease in spasticity. It is as yet unclear what the actual value of this medication is.

Selective nerve blocks, either of the tiny nerves in the muscle, of peripheral nerves, or of the nerve roots near the spinal cord can be used to control spasticity. Generally, this is useful in a person with an incomplete injury who is ambulatory and who has a muscle imbalance which interferes with ambulation. For these people, block of a single branch of a peripheral nerve can significantly improve the gait and decrease the energy needed to walk properly.

AUTONOMIC DYSREFLEXIA

In order to keep the body at the right temperature and maintain the blood pressure within normal range, blood flow through the tiny vessels all over the body is regulated in an ever-changing fashion by the autonomic nervous system. The autonomic nervous system is a series of nerves which run both inside and outside the spinal cord in a complex system of feedback controlled by the spinal cord and the brain. Spinal cord injury can affect the body's ability to control temperature and blood pressure because nerve impulses from the brain get "blocked" before they reach the part of the body below the level of the injury for which they were intended. This sets off a reaction of confused messages by the blocked nervous system and can lead to a very serious condition called *autonomic dysreflexia*.

Autonomic dysreflexia is a possible complication for anyone with an injury above T10 and is most likely to occur in someone with a cervical injury (i.e., quadriplegia). It is caused by the presence of some kind of irritation below the level of injury. By far the most common cause of autonomic dysreflexia is bladder distention and other urinary complications. Other causes include bowel impaction, pressure sores, or anything that would have produced irritation or discomfort to the body below the level of injury. In women, especially those with quadriplegia, menstruation will sometimes trigger an episode of autonomic dysreflexia. Childbirth can also be complicated by autonomic dysreflexia if it is not anticipated and appropriate precautions taken. It is important to discuss this problem with your obstetrician, so that appropriate simple measures can be taken to prevent this complication.

Symptoms of autonomic dysreflexia include severe headaches, sweating above the level of your lesion, changes in your skin (goosebumps or changes in coloring), and feelings of congestion. Some people can sense the onset of autonomic dysreflexia before these symptoms in that they have a vague, unexplainable sense that something is wrong. If you experience these symptoms and are in an at-risk group (T8 and above; with high-level lesions, particularly above T5, being most susceptible), the following steps should be taken:

1. Maintain a sitting or semireclining position if possible.
2. Check for bladder distention and quickly relieve the cause of obstruction (kinked catheter, twisted condom, plugged system, etc.).
3. Take off the shoes and check the lower extremities for other areas of irritation (tight leg bag straps, binding underwear, tight shoes, etc.).

4. Carefully, using a finger well lubricated with anesthetic jelly, check the rectum; if it is full of stool, do not evacuate the stool until you have attained control of the blood pressure using the medication prescribed by your doctor for this purpose (this may include Nifedipine, Nitropaste, Phenoxybenzamine, or others).
5. When blood pressure is under control, carefully evacuate the rectum using large amounts of xylocaine jelly and carefully monitor the blood pressure.
6. If these measures fail or if the blood pressure rises again, you should go to the hospital or SCI clinic and be evaluated and treated immediately by a physician. It is important for you to know that not all health care professionals understand the cause, the symptoms, and the treatment of autonomic dysreflexia. Therefore, if you're at risk for autonomic dysreflexia you should carry a card which explains this problem, outlines its treatment, and has the names of your SCI physicians who understand this problem and who can assist other health care professionals in treating you.

Autonomic dysreflexia can be life-threatening if it is not attended to promptly. Usually, however, it can be avoided, and it is very rare that people need to be hospitalized for this problem once they have learned how to manage it.

SUMMARY

The concepts outlined in this chapter are complex and can be confusing. Furthermore, because the management of these problems depends most importantly upon the subjective experiences and judgment of the spinal cord–injured person, it is vital that everyone with a spinal cord injury understands pain, spasticity, and autonomic dysreflexia as it may relate to his or her particular condition. When your body is doing things which you do not understand and cannot control, your level of anxiety will often increase significantly, and the increased anxiety level will in turn make the problem worse, especially in the case of the three problems discussed in this chapter. Therefore, it is very important for you to become an educated and assertive consumer. If there is something happening with your body that you do not understand or do not know how to interpret, it is important that you do whatever is necessary to gain an understanding of what is happening to you so that you can correctly interpret the messages your body is giving you and can therefore take care of yourself properly.

CHAPTER 12

Sex and Intimacy

Mark N. Ozer and Lynn Phillips

One of the most rewarding aspects of life to many people is the ability to share tenderness and intimacy with another individual. An integral part of intimacy often is a sexual relationship.

Sex, sexuality, and intimacy are all closely related topics, each with many different aspects. Emotional satisfaction, reproductive function, physical performance, physical attractiveness to other people, and establishment of relationships with others all fall to some degree or other under the general heading of sex and intimacy. The degree of importance we place on each of these issues is an intensely personal decision and one that is affected by our upbringing and other influences in our lives.

A full, satisfying sex life is just as possible after a spinal cord injury as it was before. Almost every aspect of sex, sexuality, and intimacy will remain essentially the same as before injury, even though the means toward achieving some of those goals will need to be modified. The most important aspect about sex after spinal cord injury, as it was with sex *before* spinal cord injury, is to maintain an open mind about options and be willing to try new approaches.

HOW THE SYSTEM WORKS

Sex and procreation are the means by which every species on earth is perpetuated. For most species, sex is an instinctive

147

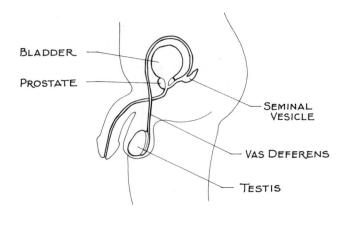

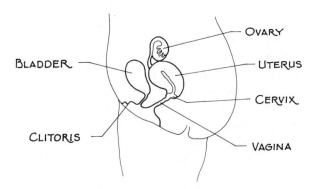

FIG. 12.1.   Male and female reproductive organs.

behavior that leads to offspring. Human reproductive behavior, however, is considerably more complex. In addition to some cultural expectations of sex, which tend to incorporate romance, love, and lust with the act of procreation, human sexual response includes arousal by sensory stimuli—sight, sound, touch, taste, smell—and erotic processes in addition to direct physical stimulation of the genitals (Fig. 12.1).

The human body has two kinds of responses to sexual stimuli—*psychogenic* (response to ''sexy'' stimuli such as erotic photographs or fantasies) and *reflexogenic* (response to direct physical stimulation). Both contribute to the body's physiological response, which in men is evidenced by penile erection and in women by enlargement of the clitoris. The nerves that control the process of erection in the male are the same as those that cause clitoral engorgement in the female, and they arise from two parts of the spinal cord. One set, the *sympathetic* nerves, come from the lower thoracic and upper lumbar cord. The *parasympathetic* nerves come from the lower sacral portion of the spinal cord. Still another nerve carries sensory input—touch and other stimuli—so that these organs are sensitive, and this nerve goes into the sacral portion of the cord.

After a spinal cord injury, as we have learned in other chapters, the body goes into a period called spinal shock when all muscles below the level of injury are flaccid. In the weeks and months after the injury, however, reflex actions and some other physical functions will return, depending upon the severity and location of the injury.

For many men the ability to have an erection will return once the body has recovered from spinal shock. The ability to have both psychogenic and reflexogenic erections is most likely in those with incomplete injuries. Many males with complete lesions are able to experience reflexogenic erections, although not psychogenic ones.

An indication of the completeness of a lesion is the absence of response to a pinprick or light touch in the area of the penis or scrotum in men, the external genitalia in women, or feelings in anal skin, and absence of conscious control of the anal sphincter in both sexes. The presence of either of these two—sensation or conscious motor control—indicates that the lesion is incomplete.

For men with incomplete lesions, that is, with some connection remaining between the brain and the spinal cord, erections are possible by both psychogenic and external stimulation as they had been prior to injury. Females are able to have intercourse regardless of the level of injury, although additional lubrication may be needed if your body does not appear to be providing the natural lubrication necessary for ease of intercourse.

EMISSION, EJACULATION, AND ORGASM IN MEN

Thus far in our discussion the process of sexual arousal has been the function of nerves coming out of the spinal cord that are called *parasympathetic*. The actual process by which sperm are carried out in fluid and deposited in the vagina so as to cause fertilization is a function of two additional sets of nerves.

The seminal emission phase is the first step in the sequence that leads to orgasmic experience. During this phase sperm stored in the ducts leading from the testes where sperm are made come up to the area within the penis where they are mixed with fluid from the prostate and other organs. The seminal fluid is thus made ready for the actual step of being propelled forward.

One other step is necessary before ejaculation can occur and the egg of the female can be fertilized. The urinary bladder must be closed so that the sperm will go forward out of the penis. The accumulation of fluid and the closure of the bladder neck are the result of the actions of the *sympathetic* nerves coming out of the lower thoracic and upper lumbar portions of the spinal cord. The actual process of propelling the semen forward is called ejaculation. This step is controlled by muscles including the *bulbocavernosus* muscle.

Orgasm is the term given for the feelings a person experiences associated with the process of emission and ejaculation and are not necessarily always the same as the muscle action. For example, some persons can experience orgasm without ejaculation having occurred and vice versa.

The retention of either some sensory or motor function adds even more to the likelihood of semen actually coming out of the penis and being ejaculated. Just as with the process of erection, those with incomplete lesions do better in general than those with complete disconnection. Although the likelihood of erection is quite high, those same persons with upper motor neuron lesions are less likely to have emission and ejaculation. The likelihood of both erection and emission leading to ejaculation is greater with spinal cord lesions low in the spinal cord.

The nerves responsible for the movement of fluid carrying the sperm or semen (sympathetic nerves) arise from the spinal cord in the thoracic and lumbar portions of the cord. A lesion in the spinal cord below the level of the sympathetic outflow but above the level of the sacral cord enables these nerves to remain under the control of the brain, because they have already left the spinal cord and can thus escape the effects of disconnection. Intact sympathetic nerves going to the area of the genitals permit continued psychogenic erections as well as seminal emission, even in those whose injury is complete.

For those far fewer men with spinal cord injury at the lowest end of the spinal cord, the effects are different. In those lower motor neuron lesions there is an increased opportunity for those having erections to continue to have them on a psychogenic basis. For those who do have erections, they are also more likely to have successful coitus and ejaculation.

In general, one may expect a greater degree of psychogenic erections with lower lesions as well as greater likelihood of seminal emission during coitus. As with all statistics dealing with sexual function, what is important is the individual characteristics of the person with injury: his degree of incompleteness; his specific level of injury; and to a considerable degree, the skill and caring of a partner.

AROUSAL, FUNCTION, AND ORGASM IN WOMEN

From a purely physiological perspective, the effects of a spinal cord injury on a woman vary considerably from those of a man. Culturally and personally, too, it is likely that a woman with spinal cord injury will experience thoughts and reactions to her sexuality quite differently from those of men with similar injuries.

Arousal for many women often has incorporated much more than direct stimulation of the clitoris and vagina. Stimulation of the breasts, neck, shoulders, and earlobes, for example, is as pleasing to many women as direct stimulation of the genital area. Consequently, actual sexual experience and participation in a sexual encounter will not change as dramatically for a woman after a spinal cord injury as it will for a man, whose ability to have and maintain erections may be affected.

Due to the female "role" in intercourse, as well, women are somewhat at an advantage since the ability to accept the penis during intercourse is not affected. As mentioned earlier, any difficulty in lessened lubrication can be remedied through the use of a lubricant such as KY jelly. And, as with men, the ability to experience orgasm varies from woman to woman, depending on the level and severity of her spinal injury.

SEXUAL ENJOYMENT

Physical function is only one aspect of sexual activity and sexual fulfillment. Many people are concerned about how sex will "feel" after injury, whether it will be satisfying for them, and whether it will be satisfying for their partners.

People who have incomplete spinal cord lesions may retain some sensation in their genital areas. Others experience heightened sensation in other parts of their bodies, such as the nipples, the skin at the level of the injury, or the earlobes. As with any sexual relationship, the best way to find out what feels good to you is to experiment with various kinds of touching.

Whether or not your partner feels "satisfied" also depends upon many factors other than whether intercourse is possible. Foreplay is an integral part of most sexual relationships because it provides sexual satisfaction and fulfillment. The same sexual activities that you enjoyed before your injury probably will be enjoyable now, and can be modified with a little creativity to be even more enjoyable. Several excellent books have been developed on the topic of sex after spinal cord injury, and they are included as resources in the listing at the end of this chapter.

REPRODUCTIVE FUNCTION IN WOMEN

Spinal cord injury most often occurs to people between the ages of 16 and 25. Consequently, a major concern for many people after injury is: Will I be able to have children?

Spinal cord injury does not affect a female's ability to have children. Although menstrual periods generally will cease for several months after injury, ovulation can continue and you may become pregnant. Consequently, women with spinal cord injuries will need to consider birth control methods if they do not wish to become pregnant. The contraceptive alternatives available are the same as those that were used before injury. However, many women find that a diaphragm is difficult to use after injury because the vaginal muscles that helped to maintain its proper position are weakened. You should discuss with your doctor which contraceptive would work best for you.

If you decide that you would like to become pregnant, you may want to talk to your physician first to discuss the best way to care for yourself and your baby throughout your pregnancy. Like all pregnant women, you will need to pay special attention to what you eat and the kinds of activities you undertake. Women with spinal cord injuries often give birth prematurely, so you should be aware of that possibility. In addition, special attention to your bowel and bladder function is essential during pregnancy.

Many women with spinal cord injuries are able to deliver their babies vaginally; others require cesarean sections. Again, discussing these options with your physician before you become pregnant will enable you to make sound decisions that are best for you.

REPRODUCTIVE FUNCTION IN MEN

Whether or not a male will be able to father children after a spinal cord injury depends on a number of factors. Those who are able to have erections and to ejaculate are most likely to be successful in impregnating their partners. However, lack of those capabilities does not necessarily mean that you will be unable to father a child. Just as a female continues to produce eggs after spinal cord injury, a male will continue to produce sperm. The problem is that the sperm must come into contact with the female partner's egg and must be sufficiently "aggressive" to fertilize the egg.

Many men with spinal cord injury have a relatively low sperm count and sperm that are not as "active" as before injury. These factors, referred to as *sperm mobility and motility,* combined with the difficulty that many men have in ejaculating after a spinal cord injury, decrease the likelihood that a spinal cord–injured man will impregnate his spouse.

Several spinal cord injury centers have developed techniques to stimulate ejaculation through the use of electrical probes, and to collect the sperm for artificial insemination of the spouse. While the success of this approach, called *electroejaculation,* is not yet established, it is an alternative that can be tried by couples who are interested in having children. You may wish to discuss this approach with your doctor if you desire to father children with your own sperm. Other parenting alternatives available include insemination of the wife from a donor's sperm and adoption.

In the years following the return of World War II spinal cord–injured veterans, many adoption agencies were unwilling to allow individuals with disabilities to adopt children, believing (wrongly) that a disability would interfere with their parenting ability and with the psychological health of their adopted children. Fortunately, these attitudes have dissipated and their validity has been completely disputed by several recent studies. More information on parenting after a spinal cord injury can be found in the resources listed at the end of this chapter.

POSSIBLE CONCERNS

When you and your partner first initiate lovemaking after one of you has sustained a spinal cord injury, you may be uncertain about how your body will respond to direct stimulation, to erotic thoughts, and to intercourse. You may have worries about the physical attractiveness of your body to your partner. You may also have concerns about what to do with the urinary catheter, for instance, or about inadvertently hurting each other. All of these concerns can lead to anxiety, discomfort, and embarrassment, none of which enhances a sexual relationship.

Sex is one of the most intimate forms of human communication, and it also is an area in which most of us feel very vulnerable. ''Performance anxiety'' is not unique to someone with a spinal cord injury, and that is an important fact to remember.

If your sexual partner is a spouse or someone with whom you have shared a close, loving relationship for a period of years or months, you may already have an intimate enough relationship so that you will feel free to discuss what your fears and concerns may be. If you are involved in a relatively new relationship, or one where discussing intimate topics is not very easy, it may be a little more difficult to bring up some of these topics. And, if you are not now involved in a sexual relationship but would like to have those kinds of relationships in the future, you may be wondering how potential sexual partners will react to you.

GETTING TO KNOW YOUR BODY

Once your body is no longer in spinal shock, you will begin to get back reflex activities and in many cases some sensation. Although your doctors will be able to give you clinical descriptions about your injury, the best way to find out what you can feel, how your body reacts to touch, or how certain parts of your body function is to get to know your own body. Although some people feel shy or otherwise embarrassed about touching themselves, the better you know your own body, the more comfortable you will feel interacting with a sexual partner and letting him/her know what gives you pleasure.

ATTITUDES

Another concern of many people after a spinal cord injury is whether people will find them sexually attractive. Sexual attractiveness comes as much from how you feel about yourself and how you project yourself to others as it does from any particular physical characteristics. This was just as true before your injury as it is today. If you think about what you find attractive about certain people, you probably will conclude that you consider many factors—personality, sensitivity, intellect, sense of humor, values, self-confidence, and physical appearance—as part of their attractiveness to you. The most difficult hurdle you probably will have to cross is convincing yourself of that fact.

Many people with spinal cord injuries are involved in happy marriage relationships or other long-term, committed relationships. Others enjoy "playing the field." Still others find themselves shying away from any intimate kind of relationship. The point is, the variety and quality of relationships "available" to you after a spinal cord injury are the same as those "available" to you before your injury. If you found it difficult to meet people before your injury, you will find it difficult meeting them now. If you are a gregarious, likable person who makes friends easily, a wheelchair and a spinal cord injury won't change that aspect of your personality. An old truism is that "The sexiest organ in the human body is the brain," and like many truisms, it has its basis in fact.

THE MECHANICS OF SEX

Perhaps the most notable difference between "preinjury" and "postinjury" sex is actual physical function and the presence of equipment—urinary catheters, braces, or hand splints, for example—that contribute to a different physical setting. As mentioned earlier, the better you understand your body, the easier it will be to convey your interests and desires to your partner. If, for example, you are a male who is able to have erections as a result of physical stimulation to the genital area, you will need to indicate to your partner how to stroke you so that you can have an erection and/or feel certain kinds of sensations. You also may have developed "sexy" sensations in other parts of your body. For your partner to be able to provide you with that pleasure, you need to be able to convey that information. Again, communication with your partner is the best way to ensure that both of you are having a pleasurable experience.

Some concerns about the "mechanics" of sex after an injury relate to possible injury or infection that might occur as a result of lovemaking. Specific concerns that have been expressed by spinal cord–injured persons and their partners include:

- *What to do with an indwelling urinary catheter*. Catheters can be left in place or removed during intercourse. Women should have no difficulty as the catheter is not located near the vagina. Men may bend the catheter alongside the penis for intercourse.
- *How to avoid urination during intercourse*. It is best to limit liquids if you think you will be having intercourse

in the next few hours. Right before you begin lovemaking, you may want to empty your bladder to minimize the possibility of urinating. Also, you can place a towel underneath you for added protection.

- *How to avoid bowel movements*. By establishing a regular bowel program (Chapter 9) you should be able to minimize the likelihood of this occurring.

- *Reducing the chance of infection when bacteria are present in the bladder*. Bladder infections can be transmitted through sexual contact, so it is wise to use a condom if you wish to have intercourse when one or both partners has a bladder infection.

ADAPTIVE AIDS

Many people use adaptive aids during sexual play. Vibrators, dildos, exotic oils, creams, and aphrodisiac potions have been a part of sex play for people in various cultures, including ours, throughout history. While some people feel uncomfortable with the idea of using such aids, others find them to be fun and sensuous additions to their lovemaking. You may wish to consider some of them as adjuncts to your sexual experiences.

Some men who are unable to have erections find that they place great importance on this particular physical function and have a strong desire to be able to have erections. If you find the inability to have erections to be a serious problem for you in sexual relationships, you may wish to consider undergoing a surgical procedure to have a *penile prosthesis* implanted. These allow you to have an erection through the placement of rods or inflatable tubes in your penis. If you are interested in the possibility of such a procedure, talk to your urologist for further information. While penile implants can give you the ability to have erections, they do not restore sensation in the genital area, and complications and infection can occur, as with any other surgical procedure.

SUMMARY

Sex and sexuality can be important aspects of one's life, and development of a close relationship that includes sex can be one of the most rewarding parts of life. A disability need not prevent you from achieving those goals. The means to achieving them may change, but that can be true for anyone, whether male or female, "disabled" or "able-bodied." Whatever techniques and psychological approaches work best for you are the "right" ones. Once you feel comfortable with your body and yourself, sexual fulfillment can be an integral part of your life and that of the person you love.

SUGGESTED READINGS

Becker, E. (1978): *Female Sexuality Following Spinal Cord Injury.* Accent Special Publications, Cheever Publishing, Inc., P.O. Box 700, Bloomington, IL 61701.

Bregman, S.: *Sexuality and the Spinal Cord Injured Woman.* Sister Kenny Institute, Dept. 188, 1800 Chicago Ave., Minneapolis, MN 55404.

Eisenberg, M. G., and Rustad, L. C.: *Sex and the Spinal Cord Injured: Some Questions and Answers.* Veterans Administration Medical Center, Cleveland, OH. Available through Superintendent of Documents, U.S. Government Printing Office, Washington, DC 20402.

Gregory, M. F. (1974): *Sexual Adjustment: A Guide for the Spinal Cord Injured.* Accent on Living Publications, Accent on Living Inc., P.O. Box 726, Bloomington, IL 61701.

Intimacy and Disability. Available from NARIC, 4407 8th Street, N.E., Washington, DC 20017.

Mooney, T., Cole, T., and Chilgren, R. (1975): *Sexual Options for Paraplegics and Quadriplegics.* Little, Brown and Co., Boston, MA.

Neistadt, M., and Baker, M. (1977): *Choices: A Sexual Guide for the Physically Disabled.* Massachusetts Rehabilitation Hospital, 125 Nashua St., Boston, MA 02114.

Rabin, B. J. (1979): *The Sensuous Wheeler: Sexual Adjustment for the Spinal Cord Injured.* Multi Media Resource Center, 1525 Franklin St., San Francisco, CA 94109.

Sex and the Disabled Female. Accent on Living, P.O. Box 700, Bloomington, IL 61701.

Sex and the Spinal Cord Injured Male. Accent on Living, P.O. Box 700, Bloomington, IL 61701.

Taggie, J., and Manley, M. S. (1978): *A Handbook on Sexuality After Spinal*

Cord Injury. Available through M. Scott Manley, 3425 So. Clarkson, Englewood, CO 80110.

Who Cares? A Handbook on Sex Education and Counseling Services for Disabled People (1979). Sex and Disability Project, George Washington University, Washington, DC.

CHAPTER 13

Sports and Recreation

Peter Axelson

Sports and recreation have always been a part of my life. Before my spinal cord injury, skiing, ice hockey, and tennis were a primary means for me to express myself physically, intellectually, and spiritually in the outdoors which I loved. I played these sports competitively, with my family and friends, and, in the case of skiing, I could also enjoy its challenges all by myself.

After my injury in 1975, I needed and sought out the comradeship of others who had spinal cord injuries. I wanted to compete in sports with my peers. As I traveled with other people in wheelchairs for sports training and competition, I learned important lessons about how to live with my disability. Eventually, however, I wanted to participate again in recreation with my family and friends who did not have physical disabilities—which was easier said than done. Yet I longed for it enough that eventually I began to find ways to achieve it.

As an engineer and product designer I looked for ways to adapt and modify recreational equipment. I ended up designing whole new devices and systems which would enable me to play with people both with and without disabilities. One such device was the ARROYA sit-ski, a composite shell with edges that not only enabled me to ski again with family and friends but permitted other people—with and without disabilities—to compete in a new recreational activity.

Although I've enjoyed designing and building adaptive equipment, I must admit that my personal goal has always been to utilize a minimum of such equipment. Ocean kayaking is one of my favorite sports—the only modification to the kayak is a molded seat in which I sit.

THE NEED FOR RECREATION

Recreation is the refreshment of body, mind, and spirit in the form of play, amusement, or relaxation.

Unfortunately, recreation is often included at the rehabilitation center as a form of passive entertainment. Barriers always exist between the viewer and the activity when recreation is nonparticipatory. When the entertainment stimulus is taken away—when the televised tennis match is over—the individual may or may not have the motivation to seek further involvement with that activity.

Being a spectator does not promote active development of recreational skills. Unlike passive viewing, when you work to learn such skills you become involved physically and intellectually. Excitement builds as you develop recreational skills which can be used throughout your life.

Through the use of adaptive equipment and/or rule modifications, many recreational activities invite participation of (and/or direct competition with) both disabled and able-bodied players. These activities do a great deal to break down social barriers between the two groups. If archery is your sport, an able-bodied archer is likely to relate to you as a fellow archer, rather than as "handicapped." Your similarities are more obvious than your differences, making it easier to relate to each other.

The psychological benefits of sports and recreation can be immense. Time and time again I witness people with spinal cord injuries who discover the excitement and fulfillment of getting out into the snow. The not-so-thrilling aspects of life suddenly become a whole lot more meaningful. My physical strength and education have taken a very rewarding direction as a direct result of my increased enthusiasm for life, which is continually enhanced through sports and recreational activity.

A SURVEY OF RECREATIONAL OPTIONS

What recreational activities did you pursue before your injury? You probably have some new physical limitations now, but otherwise you are pretty much the same person you were before. If your recreational interests are the same as before, it seems wise to consider continuing the same pursuits.

In some cases this may not be possible or may be more difficult than it is worth. If you are now paralyzed from the waist down, your pole-vaulting and tap-dancing days are probably over. However, a number of related activities are still available to you: There are numerous other track-and-field events and many styles of dance.

At the other end of the scale are sports and activities where the spinal injury does not significantly change the equipment needs of the participant or the participant's performance. Paraplegics with good sitting balance will find table tennis and pool to be as accessible as ever, requiring no unusual equipment but a wheelchair.

However, your first few games are likely to be disappointing. If you have spent some months inactive, you will find your game lacks polish, and you will have to learn to play from a seated position. At first, it may seem that your disability is a serious handicap, whereas you are actually only suffering from unfamiliarity with a new perspective. It is true that these two activities give a slight advantage to an ambulatory player (if not, everyone would play them from a chair), but the advantage is unlikely to decide a game. A good ambulatory player is not likely to beat a better, nonambulatory player.

RISK (YOU COULD GET HURT DOING IT)

People with spinal injuries are normally very aware of risk in recreation, particularly those of us who were injured during recreational activity. In general, we are more aware of the consequences of an injury than we were before we were injured. We can no longer think of accidents as things that happen to other people or exaggerate our bodies' ability to "roll with the punches."

Yet strangely enough we find more people who are willing to do our thinking for us now that we have a disability. Family, friends, and health professionals tend to steer us away from high-risk activities. Their motivation is worth examining briefly.

First, other people's disabilities bring out maternal and paternal instincts in some people. That is a polite way of saying they tend to treat us like children, and children are not qualified to make their own decisions about physical risk.

Second, other people's disabilities are seen as object lessons by some people, evidence that the world really is as dangerous as they fear (there is a story of a woman who was walking with crutches, who overheard a mother say to a child, "There. You see what happened to her when she tried to roller-skate on her toy box?"). These people disapproved of high-risk recreation all along, and now that you have given them the proof they needed, they will be happy to tell you all about it.

Third, your disability may be seen as evidence that you do not have enough sense to take care of yourself and need adult supervision. These are the people who say, "Don't you remember? That's how you got hurt," when the subject of high-risk recreation comes up. It was probably one of the more memorable experiences of your life, but these people are not totally convinced of your sanity, so they have to ask.

Fourth, people with disabilities are often perceived as physically fragile. A person who trips and falls may be seen as an object of amusement, whereas a person who falls out of a wheelchair is seen as an object of concern. Heaven forbid you should fall off a horse!

Everyone has the right to risk. Most people get great pleasure from risks challenged and overcome. With some, it can be the risk of landing on Park Place with two hotels, or the risk of Pac Man being caught by a ghost. With others, physical risk is required. Since maximum enjoyment of risk comes from a full understanding of the risk, let us look at how a spinal injury can affect physical risks.

The injured area of your back has probably been weakened. If you have had a spinal fusion in the last year, you must pay particular attention to any activity which might put unusual stresses on your spine.

If you have any paralysis in any of your limbs, you will not be able to use them as effectively to "catch yourself" as you could before. So if you should fall from a horse, an inability to use your legs will increase your chances of landing badly.

A secondary injury will have greater impact on your life. Persons who use a wheelchair may find themselves temporarily immobilized by a broken arm, while a person who walks might find it just a temporary inconvenience.

The muscles of paralyzed limbs tend to atrophy, reducing "padding" over bones and reducing circulation. For these and other reasons, the areas affected by nerve damage are more easily injured (and slower to heal) than they were before.

Specific activities will have their own specific risks and should be considered carefully in light of your current physical condition. However, physical activity, even at the price of some physical risk, is better for your body than long-term inactivity. Whatever the activity, learn the risks and know everything you can about the sport and then go for it!

RECREATION USING ADAPTIVE EQUIPMENT

A participant with a spinal injury will need more (or different) adaptive equipment than was needed before the injury.

Three- or four-track skiing, sit-skiing, and specialized leg prostheses for amputees who rock climb are examples of how adaptive equipment can promote integrated participation. In the case of competitive sports, rules often need to be modified to keep scoring balanced with level of ability, or people with similar disabilities will have to be matched against each other. Many people are unwilling to participate in recreational activities under these terms. Others find them quite acceptable. Let us examine the common reasons for nonparticipation.

1. Adaptive equipment is required; therefore the recreation is not the "real thing."

This is a common complaint, but it overlooks one important point. Nearly all sporting activities require adaptive equipment, even for the participants without disabilities. For thousands of years, people have been using these types of equipment to extend their abilities beyond the limitations of their bodies. Because these needs are commonplace, we tend to ignore them. It is a case of not seeing the forest for the trees.

A baseball glove is a piece of adaptive equipment. It is worn to compensate for the player's small, soft hands which in their unprotected state are simply not capable of dealing with solidly hit baseballs. Since this is the norm, we fail to notice it.

Many quadriplegics cannot grip a standard cue firmly enough to play pool. Some put Velcro straps on their pool cues, and some choose not to play the game rather than play with "adaptive equipment." Actually, everyone plays pool with adaptive equipment, since everyone plays with some sort of a cue.

The game of basketball requires basketball courts, basketball nets, and basketballs. Wheelchair basketball requires the same equipment, plus wheelchairs. Skiing requires skis. Some disabled skiers need specialized equipment, such as sit-skis, but no one is so "able-bodied" as to eliminate the need for skis. A few skiers may express sympathy toward you, since you "can't really ski" or "can't ski without equipment," quite oblivious to the fact that all skiers suffer from the same limitation.

I am a pilot. I have slightly different needs than a pilot without a disability, but we both need wings.

2. Rule modifications are required, so the recreation is not the "real thing."

This argument is similar to the equipment argument. Rules will be required in any case. A good set of rules makes a game difficult enough to be challenging, but not so difficult as to be discouraging.

The rules of tennis and the size of a tennis court varied in the early days of the sport. Over the years, experience showed how much area the average person could be expected to defend, given one bounce of the tennis ball. If not for the speed, maneuverability, and reach limitations which we call "normal," we could dispense with the bounce.

If we had the speed of cheetahs, and the arm of gorillas, no-bounce tennis would be an exciting and challenging sport. But with human beings, no-bounce tennis would be boring to play and to watch; few serves would be returned and long volleys would only occur during noncompetitive "exhibition games."

Allowing the ball to bounce adds interest and excitement to the game, and by making the objective achievable (hit the ball back over the net before the ball hits the ground a second time), the players can develop skill and confidence.

To achieve this same level of interest and excitement in wheelchair tennis, two bounces are allowed. People in wheelchairs have even greater physical limitations than able-bodied people, at least as far as the sport of tennis is concerned. Because of the seated position, reach is reduced. Because of the added weight of the wheelchair and because arm muscles are not as effective as leg muscles, accleration is reduced. With a simple rule change (hit the ball back before it hits the ground a third time), wheelchair tennis becomes an equivalent challenge to "stand-up" tennis.

3. Scoring is segregated by physical ability, so the competition is "unreal."

In most competitive sports, the object is to do the best you can within your physical limitations. To test their progress, people challenge other people with similar abilities.

In many sports, this means a person's choice of competitors is limited because to play against someone whose abilities and skills are radically different from one's own (whether greater or lesser) does not give one the opportunity to test or develop one's own skills. To simplify the process of finding compatible competition, these sports people are broken into categories by whatever scale is appropriate. Some common measures are size, age, experience, and sex. Middleweight boxers are not asked to fight heavyweight boxers, high school football teams do not play college teams, novice hang glider pilots are scored separately from masters, male gymnasts are not expected to compete against females. In all these examples, if they chose to compete, they would expect to lose and would not find the experience rewarding. Neither would their competitors who would expect to win.

Physical disabilities are common enough that many sports have classifications according to disability. Often these are based on "level of injury." In the case of spinal injuries, the level is determined by muscle function, rather than the actual point of damage. In such sports as competitive swimming or track events, competing against people with similar abilities will give a more accurate assessment of personal achievement than would competition against people with greater (or lesser) abilities. An interesting sidelight to this is the changing state of wheelchair road racing. In the last 10 years, a number of wheelchair marathons have been run in conjunction with running marathons (including the Boston Marathon since 1977). In the beginning, the fastest wheelchair racers were significantly slower than the fastest runners. Since then, great advances have been made in technology and technique. As improvements in footgear and training have brought "normal" marathon times to levels unachieveable by the ancient Greeks, aluminum frames and lowered seats have brought wheelchair marathon times to levels unachievable 10 years ago.

Currently, the fastest wheelchair racers are significantly faster than the fastest runners. It would hardly be fair to athletes without disabilities if they were forced to compete in marathons against wheelchair athletes.

4. Lessened ability means lesser challenges.

If your feelings of accomplishment are based on how you were, rather than how you are, this may be a problem. Anyone who lives long enough will have to face the fact that they can no longer do some things as well as before. If you are a climber and now have limited use of your legs, you will probably be climbing shallower walls than before. You will not find them any less challenging.

The goal of climbing is not simply to get to the top. It is common to find a party of climbers struggling up one side of a mountain, while on the other side, a road goes to the summit. Challenges are where you find them and how you define them.

5. All the same reasons the able-bodied have.

Recreation is a waste of time; it is more important to get some more work done; I don't know how to get started; recreation is for "beautiful people"; people will look at me; it's too difficult; it's too much work; it's too expensive; it's too dangerous; you can't teach an old dog new tricks; I can turn on the TV and see professionals doing it better than I ever could; I don't have any place to keep the equipment; I'm too shy; I don't know if I'm really going to enjoy it; I'm too success-oriented; I heard about a guy who was exercising and he dropped dead of a heart attack, just like that—I think I'll have another beer.

These reasons are just as valid now as they were then.

NEW RECREATIONAL ACTIVITIES

You may wish to supplement your old pursuits with some new recreational activities, or you may be ready to put old pursuits behind you and start fresh. Getting back on the horse that threw you will give you confidence, or get you trampled. Now that you have had time to think about it, you may find the ratio of regard to risk is not high enough to entice you back. If you injured your spine while cliff-diving at Acapulco, you may be ready to consider a new hobby.

Following is an assortment of recreational activities. This is a very small sample, and each activity is given only a brief glance, but it will give you an idea of the things that are available.

ARCHERY

Use of legs is not important in this sport. A standing archer has a slight advantage over a seated archer because of the slight difference in height, but a seated archer may be slightly more stable. Out of fairness to your friends who stand (and in compliance with NWAA competition rules), you should not brace your shoulder or arm on your chair.

People with higher injuries and reduced hand strength will find a variety of accessories to assist them. The simplest is a strap which helps hold the bow in the archer's hand. Another is a "hook on a handle" which allows the archer to draw the bow without gripping the bowstring.

Bows come in all weights and sizes, and can accommodate most people's reach and strength. Crossbows can be used by people with limited arm movement or by people who simply prefer crossbows. A crossbow is a bow mounted horizontally on a stock, similar to a rifle. The bow is cocked, an arrow (called a "bolt") placed on the stock, and the string is released by pulling a trigger. Most of the accessories that would apply to a rifle (such as mounts and scopes) can be used with a crossbow.

BASKETBALL

Wheelchair basketball started under the guidance of the Veterans Administration when the boys came home from World War II. In 1949, the National Wheelchair Basketball Association was formed. The game is now played worldwide, with over 150 teams in the United State, seasonal competition, and regional and national tournaments.

The first "sport wheelchairs" were built for basketball, and a great deal of modern wheelchair design grew from what worked well on the basketball court.

The rules are quite similar to conventional basketball. A player cannot take more than two pushes while possessing the ball just as his conventional counterpart cannot take more than two steps. The chair is considered part of the player and the usual rules of blocking apply, whether done with an elbow or a wheel. One dissimilarity is the "physical advantage foul."

To keep play balanced and interesting, all players are required to stay in their seats. Otherwise a person with a low injury could stand during passing or shooting, suddenly becoming 2 feet taller than the competition. Not fair. Even if you have some use of your legs, you are not allowed to use them. This may seem a bit artificial, but it is common in sports. Players are often forbidden to do things they are physically capable of (such as holding a soccer ball or hitting below the belt) to make sports safer or more interesting. A violation of this rule is a physical advantage foul. Your opponent gets a free throw, and if you earn three of these fouls, you're out of the game.

Players are broken into three categories. Class I is people with complete spinal paraplegia at T9 or above (or comparable disability), Class II is with spinal paraplegia at T10 or below (or comparable disability), and Class III is all other disabilities. Players are given value points equal to their calls. A team can be made of any combination of players, providing the players on the court do not have total value points greater than 12.

Wheelchair basketball is exciting to play, and to watch. It does have one characteristic which is common in wheelchair sports: People without disabilities are not allowed to play, at least not in the United States. Why not? With the personal advantage foul rule in place, what is the difference between a Class III player and a player with no disability? From the standpoint of competition, there is no difference. The issue is an emotional one, with strong feelings and strong arguments both for and against. In sports, should wheelchairs be seen as devices for the disabled or as recreational equipment for anyone?

BOATING

Sailing offers a range of activities, from the relaxation of simply sailing about to the competition of racing. As very little walking around is done on small boats, low spinal injuries should not present much difficulty, and a sailor may choose to compete against sailors without disabilities in a variety of one-design classes.

The intensity of one-design racing (where the competitors sail identical boats) has to be seen to be believed. If you are tired of "special treatment" because you are using a wheelchair, just wait for the starting gun of a Hobie 16 race.

A catamaran has many advantages over monohull boats. Catamarans have a fabric "trampoline" between the hulls. To sail them well, considerable upper body strength is required, but for a sailor who is paralyzed from the waist down, no equipment modifications are needed. You may wish to make some modifications to suit your personal tastes, such as tiller position and pulley placement, but so might anyone else.

It is recommended that either the boat or the sailor be padded. This can be accomplished by wearing a wet suit. Zippers can be installed to make the suit easier to put on and take off. Padding can be added around bony prominences to more evenly distribute weight while sitting. Bare feet are not advisable since toes could be easily damage by ropes and fittings.

Power boating, canoeing, white-water rafting are all available to people with spinal cord injuries. You may have to modify techniques, such as paddle stroke, to take advantage of your abilities. You may also need to modify your sitting position. In a canoe, large foam pads on each side of your legs may help hold you securely. *Do not* strap yourself into a boat; it could be dangerous in event of a capsize. Personal floatation devices are important safety items. If you have had shifts of fat and muscle tissue since your injury, your buoyancy will be affected. Test your life jacket (or other such device) in a swimming pool to be sure it will float you with your head out of water.

CYCLING

From the standpoint of passenger miles for a given amount of energy, the bicycle is the most efficient form of transportation. Bicycles propelled by leg muscles have been used for years. The advent of a hand-powered bicycle was supported by the Veterans Administration Rehabilitation R&D Program. Front-wheel drive simplified the design problem. The cyclist holds two cranks, powers the bike by rotating the cranks, and steers by moving the cranks from side to side. At low speed or at a stop, outrigger wheels keep the bike from falling over. To brake, the cyclist backpedals (like a conventional bicycle with coaster brake).

Like conventional bicycling, riding is more difficult to describe than to perform. A person with good upper-body strength can learn to ride quite quickly. For extended traveling, a handcycle is considerably faster than a wheelchair.

Another device is the Unicycle, which attaches to the front

of a wheelchair, converting it temporarily into a front-wheel drive, hand-powered tricycle. It is powered and steered like the handbike. The Unicycle has the advantage of three-wheel stability, and it can be removed quickly at the rider's destination.

This sport gives good exercise and the ability to integrate with other cyclists, but it is not without hazards. By zipping around at cycling speeds instead of walking speeds, an accident is likely to be more spectacular. Protective gloves and a cycling helmet are good ideas, and so is watching where you are going.

DANCING

Dancing is exercise. It also has obvious social aspects. Square dancing in wheelchairs requires a bit more room than square dancing on foot. I had the pleasure of dancing as a member of the Colorado Wheelers square dance team when I was still living in Colorado. I have also enjoyed square dancing as part of a square with dancers who do not have disabilities. Most other forms of dancing can be adapted to one's disability, if one is in pleasant company (and if one is in unpleasant company, why dance?).

FIELD EVENTS

The National Wheelchair Athletic Association sponsors field events in each of its 16 regions. The events include discus, shotput, and precision javelin.

In traditional javelin throw, points are scored for distance. In precision javelin, a target is marked on the ground. This target is a series of concentric rings, with increasing point values as the center is approached.

The NWAA classifies competitors into seven categories. Before being allowed to compete, prospective participants must have their levels of muscular function determined by a doctor or physical therapist. One need not use a wheelchair in their usual activities to compete in NWAA events, though wheelchairs are required for the events themselves.

FLYING

By observing birds, insects, and those few mammals and fish that fly, we find that use of legs is not essential to aviation. However, most of the adaptive equipment which people use to fly (such as airplanes) use foot control for steering and braking, at least while on the ground.

There are some exceptions. The Ercoupe is a light, two-person airplane which was built with a steering wheel that combines rudder and aileron controls. The only foot control is a brake pedal, which was only used on the ground and easily adapted to hand control. The Ercoupe went out of production in the 1960s, but many are available on the used aircraft market.

Low-wing airplanes are easiest to get in and out of from a wheelchair. They are also easiest for preflight inspection. A hand control is available for a number of Piper aircraft. This device clamps to one rudder pedal, allowing the pilot to steer with one lever (push for left, pull for right) instead of two pedals.

A medical certificate is required for solo flight. A student with a significant disability usually will be given a restricted medical certificate. After the student passes a flight test, a Statement of Demonstrated Ability will be issued, usually with operational limitations (e.g., valid only in aircraft equipped with hand controls).

Ultralight aircraft offer the experience of fight without the formality of medical certification, but only within certain limits. An ultralight aircraft cannot carry a passenger or fly over populated areas. For the most part, ultralight pilots risk only themselves, and so are allowed to make their own judgments regarding their fitness.

Some ultralights come equipped with hand controls, and most others can be easily modified. At least one flying club, the Tennessee Air Cooperative, owns and operates adapted ultralights for members' use.

The hazards of flying are great, but for many people, the rewards are far greater.

HIKING

For all but the easiest trails, you will need knobby tires. The indoor tread which is found on most wheelchairs will get stuck in short order if you get off onto soft ground. Suitable tires (and wheelrims, if needed) can often be found in bicycle shops.

Wheelchair hiking is more challenging than hiking on foot. Some barriers which are insignificant to a walker (such as a trail narrowing between two trees) are impassible to a wheelchair.

Others (such as fence or a fallen log) will require dismounting, climbing over or through, and pushing the chair ahead. Dealing with these obstacles calls for advanced planning and considerable familiarity with the limitations of your equipment.

If you are hiking with people without disabilities, a rope and harness may help pull you through unusually steep or soft areas. In exchange for their help, you could carry the lunch beneath your chair.

Wilderness survival has hazards for everyone, from frostbite to snakebite, and your disability may add to these hazards. As the Boy Scouts say, be prepared! If you are not familiar with the rigors of outdoor adventure, adventure with someone who is.

Practice with your equipment before going on any extended hikes. Your tent may be difficult to set up without assistance. If so, it is better to discover this in your backyard than in authentic rain-and-mosquito conditions.

RADIO-CONTROLLED MODELING

Radio-controlled modeling includes a variety of competitive sports, from off-road racing to aerobatics. The skills required are the same as for the "real thing," but since the driver or pilot is not actually in the moving vehicle, the physical risks are substantially reduced. Also, the costs are substantially reduced.

The models are controlled from a radio "sender," usually a small box with one or two joysticks (similar to another modern recreational activity, the playing of video games). A radio receiver in the car or plane (or boat or dirigible or whatever your imagination can concoct) translates signals from the sender to control commands in the model. There are hundreds of radio control clubs and contests in the United States, and thousands throughout the world. Competition is active and intense. Classes are based on the number of control channels available to the contestants. Two-channel (one single joystick) soaring contests are popular and prestigious in the radio control world.

Incidentally, there are no special competition categories for people with disabilities. If you can operate a joystick, you can compete with everyone else.

For more information, call a local hobby shop; they're listed in the yellow pages.

ROAD RACING

In the last 10 years, wheelchair road racing has become quite popular. Over these years, road-racing wheelchairs have become quite specialized. As with racing bicycles, the tires are narrow and hard, and the frames are made of lightweight alloy tubing. For minimum air resistance, the seats are low to the ground, and for higher "gearing," the pushrims are small, often as small as 1 foot in diameter.

Road racing is a relatively expensive sport because a road-racing chair is not particularly useful for anything else. After this initial purchase, training costs are low, and travel costs can be high depending on where you like to race. Many wheelchair road races (including marathons) are run in conjunction with long-distance footraces.

SKIING

I use (and was involved in the design of) the ARROYA downhill skiing system. The ARROYA prototype was an improvement over the Norwegian pulk (Norsk for sled), but it was clear that substantial design work was needed to successfully integrate skiers such as you and me into the existing sport of downhill skiing. The Veterans Administration Rehabilitation R&D Program supported the development of the ARROYA sit-ski design, which incorporates a tunnel section with four stainless steel edges that allow the skier control and maneuverability by shifting weight and by using appropriate arm movements. Sit-skis must be chairlift compatible and have a built-in evacuation harness in the event a chairlift breaks down.

Sit-skiers have been racing in slalom, giant slalom, and downhill events at the National Handicapped Ski Championships since 1980. Sit-skiing not only allows competition with other sit-skiers but allows you to ski again with family and friends. Most ski areas working with sit-skiers now recognize NHSRA certification of sit-skiers to ski untethered. The tetherer is a certified instructor who can follow behind with a line attached to assist with turning and stopping while you learn the required skills. To find the location of the nearest ski area working with sit-skiers contact the National Handicapped Sports and Recreation Association listed in Appendix 2. For skiers with good balance and trunk stability there is a monoski. This device perches the skier above a single ski to enable edge control, very similar to a three-track skier (a skier with a leg amputation balances on one ski). In fact the monoskier uses outriggers (short ski tips attached to a forearm clutch) in the same way that a three-track skier does.

SWIMMING

Swimming can be enjoyed by practically anyone, and it is great exercise. Since the swimmer's weight is supported by the water, the wheelchair and crutches can be left at poolside. Swimming can give a tremendous feeling of freedom and accomplishment.

While swimming is pleasant, drowning is not. Do not expect to be able to swim well without some retraining. Depending on your level of injury, you may have to learn to swim all over again.

People with limited leg movement may have to learn to use their arms more, and people with limited arm movement may have to learn new strokes (such as the breaststroke or an elementary backstroke). But by and large, it is easier to move in water than on land.

In competitive swimming, there are classifications for people with similar disabilities as there are in track and field events.

One interesting and exciting activity is scuba diving. Although it relies heavily on adaptive equipment (airtanks, regulators, goggles, etc.), the same equipment is needed by everyone.

TENNIS

Since its inception in the mid-1970s, wheelchair tennis has been the fastest growing wheelchair sport. It is relatively inexpensive, requiring only a tennis racquet, a wheelchair, and access to a tennis court.

Like stand-up tennis, it can be enjoyed by beginners lobbing balls back and forth, and experts can enjoy playing as though their lives depend on it. They sign contracts with sponsors, and if they feel like it, insult line judges just like "regular" tennis players.

For the serious player, there are special sport wheelchairs. These are as light as practical, with aluminum frames and no frills such as brakes. The backs are low, so as not to interfere with the player's stroke. Weighing 20 pounds less than a standard wheelchair, they make a real difference in speed and maneuverability.

The two-bounce rule does more than let wheelchair players compete against each other. By fortunate coincidence, it allows fair and competitive games to be played between people with and without disabilities. This is far more entertaining than if one form of tennis had a significant advantage, since it eliminates the need for "handicapping" (giving one player extra points at the start of the game), or slowing one player by mechanical means (if the standing players had the advantage, they could be given a backpack which weighed the same as their opponent's chair, and if the seated players had the advantage, they could take the air out of their tires).

WEIGHT LIFTING

The NWAA has chosen the bench lift as its one weight-lifting event. In this position, the lifter lays on his back (as of yet, there is no women's competition) on a horizontal bench. The barbell is placed on a rack, about 1 foot above his chest. The lifter grabs the bar, presses it upward, and holds it motionless at arm's length.

Competitor classification is by weight, not disability. A person with a low spinal injury can compete fairly in the bench lift against anyone his own size.

SELECTING APPROPRIATE ACTIVITIES

Do you have good balance, flexibility, coordination, sensation, endurance, strength, upper extremity function, mobility, range of motion, hand function, etc.? Do you have limitations due to weight or current and previous injuries? A thorough appraisal and understanding of your own functional abilities will lead to a better selection of appropriate recreation. Keep in mind that your functional abilities will progress during the rehabilitation process.

In choosing your recreational activities, it is important to examine interest and motivation factors, your own and those of other people who will participate in the recreational activity. Here are some preferences to consider:

Physical vs intellectual vs spiritual activities
Active vs passive activities
Group vs individual activities
Modified rules vs no adaptation of the activity
Competitive vs noncompetitive activities
Segregated vs integrated activities within disability
Sports requiring the use of the wheelchair or not
Socially interactive vs solitude
Creative vs activities with minimal intellectual demands

You may have the desire (1) to engage in recreational activities that are not competitive in nature and (2) to participate in integrated activities which allow recreation with family and friends.

Do not forget your emotional needs! Attention, risk, fear, exhilaration, relaxation, and excitement are some examples of emotions which you may (or may not!) wish to experience in recreational activities.

If independence is important, look for activities where you are able to be as independent as possible and are not required to rely upon other people for assistance.

WHERE TO START

Though an activity might appeal to you, you may not know how to get started in it, or perhaps you need more information to help you make up your mind. Here are a few ways to get the help you want.

Adaptive Recreation Programs

Usually a national organization can tell you about adaptive recreation programs available in your geographic location.

Instruction can be obtained through a variety of sources, including both adaptive recreation programs, community recreation programs, and university programs. For both individuals and programs, safety issues must be considered. Proper clothing, personal gear, and equipment must be selected and the special concerns of individual disabilities must be managed.

National Sporting Associations for Adapted Activity

You can ask to receive newsletters from regional or national recreation programs where adaptive devices and systems are often advertised. Universities with a physical education, special education, or adapted physical education program are a good resource. Recreation programs that do not identify themselves as providers of recreational activity for people with disabilities may be a valuable source of information on equipment as well. They may also be sponsoring activities that are barrier-free. Local sporting goods stores may be able to identify names of local clubs, groups, and organizations.

Other Resources

Other resources include national sporting associations for adapted recreational activity. Addresses of sports organizations are included in Appendix 2. In particular you want to contact the National Handicapped Sports and Recreational Association (NHSRA) and the National Wheelchair Athletic Association (NWAA).

CONTACTING NONDISABILITY RECREATION PROGRAMS

Local retail stores for sporting goods equipment often sponsor courses through their shops. Local colleges, universities, and adult education programs offer courses in a variety of recreational activities. By talking with the instructor about your particular disability, he or she may be able to incorporate you into a course. Contact magazines such as *Sports 'N Spokes*.

CONTACTING MANUFACTURERS OF ADAPTIVE EQUIPMENT

This is a sure way to obtain specific information on various recreational activities. ABLEDATA, a computerized data base which contains information on rehabilitation products and manufacturers, can be reached through the National Association for Rehabilitation Information Center (NARIC) in Washington, D.C. Once a manufacturer has been identified, you can obtain product literature and instruction manuals on adaptive equipment.

Information and instructional video tapes are often available from the manufacturer as well.

SELECTING, OBTAINING, AND MAINTAINING EQUIPMENT

Selecting, obtaining, and maintaining adaptive equipment can be both challenging and frustrating, although adaptive devices and systems can be found through a number of sources. The first places to try are the recreation department within a rehabilitation program and magazines that publish information on recreational activities.

When trying to choose among the products of several different companies, try out the equipment and if possible, talk with individuals who have used it. Determine how long the manufacturer has been in business and if the company is financially responsible. Make sure the company stands behind its product! Important considerations are durability, performance, maintenance requirements, cost, and portability for travel. Ask questions before committing yourself to purchase an item.

Once you have chosen the appropriate device or system, you may find that your budget does not allow direct purchase for your personal use. If you do not have the financial resources to purchase the equipment, you will need to do some fund raising. You can offer to put a sponsor's name on the equipment to generate publicity for the supporting institution. Many individuals and companies are willing to donate money for equipment because of the tax deduction which is available to them. Individuals can sometimes identify a source of reimbursement. Medical insurance companies are paying for adaptive equipment for recreation just as they are paying for daily living and vocational equipment to enhance an important component of your life. For veterans with disabilities, the Veterans Administration Prosthetics Service can provide information concerning adaptive equipment that is approved for purchase.

It is also possible to build your own equipment, but this can be a time-consuming project and can cost more in the long run than you would spend on commercially available equipment.

Instructional courses on the use of adaptive recreational equipment are often available. Manufacturers will often provide instructional clinics for groups of people. Contact adaptive recreation programs that are experienced with the equipment you will be using. Almost always an organization or program will be available to provide instruction on the use of a particular device or system. You may only find a handful of programs in the country and you will have to travel to that program to obtain initial instruction. Once you have the initial skills and resources you should be able to integrate into a program in your area, start a program of your own, or pursue the activity by yourself or with family and friends.

LOOKING AHEAD—THE FUTURE ROLE OF ADAPTIVE EQUIPMENT

You may have an interest in a recreational activity which is not currently enjoyed by people with spinal cord injuries. If so, you have a choice to make. You can either look for another activity or look for ways to adapt the activity yourself. It may be that no one with your ability and interest has approached the problem before.

SUMMARY

Devices and systems increase your potential for enjoying recreational activities with family and friends. It appears that participation in "special" recreation programs is no longer the only recreation a person with a disability need look forward to. There is an increased desire for participation in integrated recreational activities.

Adaptive equipment can help you to challenge barriers which often bar you from participation in recreational activity. It can help to deal with inaccessibility and liability concerns of recreation programmers. You can use equipment to promote your independence and thereby avoid the paternalism which is often associated with adaptive recreation programming. Recreational activities, in general, are utilizing more and more equipment. Access to existing recreational activities is made possible by the development of modifications to recreational equipment and by the development of new devices and systems to allow participation within existing activities.

The creation of recreational activities is on the rise. New sports utilizing adaptive equipment have been highlighted in magazines such as *Outside*. As is often the case, it will be your personal desire that can provide the motivation for new inventions and innovations. There are many opportunities to create new recreational activities that also happen to be "accessible." This is a great opportunity and challenge for rehabilitation and recreation professionals.

SUGGESTED READINGS

Elliott, B.: *Guide to the Selection of Musical Instruments with Respect to Physical Ability and Disability*. Settlement Music School, 416 Queen St., Philadelphia, PA 19147.

Lane, J., and Schaaf, D. (Eds.): *Wheelchair Bowling*. Wheelchair Bowlers of Southern California, 6512 Cadiz Circle, Huntington Beach, CA 92647.

Physical fitness: sports and recreation for those with lower limb amputation or impairment (1985). *Journal of Rehabilitation Research and Development*, Clinical Supplement No. 1. Office of Technology Transfer (153D), Veterans Administration Medical Center, 50 Irving St., N.W., Washington, DC 20422.

Sports 'N Spokes. Paralyzed Veterans of America, 5201 N. 19th Ave., Phoenix, AZ 85015.

SQUID. Handicapped Scuba Association, 1104 El Prado, San Clemente, CA 92672.

Waterskiing for the Physically Disabled. Mission Bay Aquatic Center, 1001 Santa Clara Point, San Diego, CA 92109.

CHAPTER 14

Travel and Transportation

Lynn Phillips

One aspect of "getting around" after a spinal cord injury is personal mobility. With an appropriate wheelchair, adaptive devices, and architectural alterations to your own home, it is relatively easy to make your personal environment as accessible as you want it to be. Those are the kinds of things over which you will exercise a lot of personal control, dependent only upon your resources and decisions about how many adaptations are desirable. If your bedroom is located up a flight of stairs, you will decide whether you want to install a lift, use crutches to get upstairs, move your bedroom downstairs, or move to a more accessible home. When dealing with the rest of the world, however, you don't have those kinds of personal choices. If a restaurant is located up a flight of steps, you probably will not want to eat there. Consequently, the idea of traveling and having to negotiate unknown environments from the perspective of a wheelchair user may be somewhat forbidding.

Fortunately, the world today is much more accessible to persons in wheelchairs than it was even 10 or 15 years ago. With a little planning and access to good sources of information, travel to almost any section of the United States and much of the world should be just as enjoyable from a wheelchair as it was before you became disabled.

GETTING THERE

The most common method of transportation for most of us is our own automobile. A personal automobile allows you to set your own schedule, to stop and sightsee along the way, room for storage of whatever you want to take with you, and a known, controllable environment. Those factors remain the same whether one is using a wheelchair or not. The factors that may change are the accessibility of rest stops, restaurants, and motels along the way.

Due to federal legislation mandating accessibility of public buildings, many state-run rest areas along interstate highways now have wheelchair-accessible restrooms. When such facilities are available, they usually are noted clearly on highway signs and at the rest areas themselves with the international symbol for access to the disabled (Fig. 14.1). Most states have an office for individuals with disabilities and can provide specific information about wheelchair-accessible rest areas in their state. In addition, there often is an information booth at the first rest stop you encounter when crossing state lines on the interstate system.

Service stations usually have different self-service and full-service gasoline prices. Some companies have a company policy that they will provide full service to disabled drivers at self-serve prices. Some states have state laws mandating full-service gas at self-serve prices for disabled drivers. In most places, however, such a policy is left up to the owner's discretion.

The best way to locate accessible hotels, motels, and res-

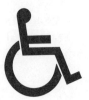

FIG. 14.1. International symbol for access by the disabled.

taurants on the road is to purchase one of the travel guides for disabled travelers listed at the end of this chapter or to contact one of the major automobile clubs, such as the American Automobile Association (AAA), which provide information about accessibility in their tour books. Roadside facilities vary significantly in the degree of accessibility provided.

Another common method of transportation today is airline travel and, in general, airline travel is becoming easier all the time for travelers with disabilities, although experiences vary widely depending upon which airline you select, which airport you use, and the personal sensitivity and understanding of airline and airport personnel. In theory, airline travel should be a relatively simple method of transportation for a traveler with disability and should pose little or no problem for airline or airport personnel. In practice, it sometimes gets a little complicated, so awareness of possible pitfalls is the best preparation for travel in the skies.

When making your reservations, always inform the reservations agent that you use a wheelchair. This will enable the agent to assist you in getting an accessible seat on the airplane and to notify ground personnel at the airports you will be flying out of and into that you will require assistance in boarding and deplaning. Most airlines ask that you arrive at the airport 1 to 2 hours before flight time to allow ample time to get you and your wheelchair onto the plane.

For airports that have jetways from the terminal to the plane, it often is possible to remain in your own wheelchair until you reach your seat on the plane. Different airlines and airports have different policies on this, so it is worth checking out the policy at your airport beforehand if keeping your own chair as long as possible is important to you. For airports that do not have jetways, i.e., those at which you must go up a flight of steps to enter the airplane, airline personnel will assist you in transferring to a "boarding chair" or "aisle chair." The most often used chair is a lightweight one with two small wheels in the back, a narrow, slightly padded seat, no arm-rests, and a tall back with a handle. It also has several safety straps to hold the occupant in place. This chair cannot be maneuvered by the individual sitting in it, so it is essential that it be used only for necessary transportation from one point to another and that airline personnel not "abandon" you in some corner of the airport while they attend to other business.

Going up and down airplane stairs in such a chair requires strong, knowledgeable airline personnel. If you feel uncomfortable about the level of capability of the people assigned to carry you up or down the stairs, request additional or alternate assistance. It is your safety and your body at stake.

If you use a powered wheelchair, you should be aware that the airlines have very strict policies about transporting batteries. Due to the hazards of fire and explosions, wet cell batteries are prohibited on many airlines. Dry or gel cell batteries are permitted. However, individuals with gel cell batteries on occasion have not been permitted to take their batteries with them because of an airline employee's ignorance about the difference between wet and gel cell batteries. Again, your own knowledge of the regulations is your best protection against someone else's lack of knowledge.

Once on board an aircraft, a wheelchair user generally is committed to staying seated during most of the flight. Most airlines do not permit you to bring your own wheelchair on board, since aisles and lavatories are not wide enough for wheelchairs. Consequently, you will need to calculate your fluid intake and bathroom needs prior to flying as you probably will be unable to use the restroom. The Boeing 767, however, does have a special on-board wheelchair, and a bathroom that is accessible with that chair.

If your trip requires changing planes at one or more airports to reach your destination, you would do well to check your wheelchair only as far as the next airport so that you can get around the airport on your own during any layovers.

Able-bodied travelers do not need to remain under the watchful eye of an airline employee, and there is no reason why you should.

While the above example may leave the impression that airline travel is more trouble than it is worth, the typical experience is one in which the passenger with a disability is treated with respect and courtesy. As airlines have become more accustomed to dealing with passengers who have disabilities, they have been improving their overall performance in this area. In all practicality, however, you may encounter a situation such as the ones described above at some point in your life if you travel a lot. Knowing that others have had similar experiences and trying to understand the basis for the problems often can serve to avoid similar situations in the future.

Train travel is possible for wheelchair users in some areas of the country. Amtrak is building its new cars and new stations to be accessible to wheelchairs, and all routes with Superliner Service (the California Zephyr, Desert Wind, and Pioneer, which serve Chicago to San Francisco, Los Angeles, and Seattle, respectively) feature special sleeping rooms that span the entire width of the train and include toilet facilities and sleeping accommodations that have been specially designed for disabled travelers. If you are interested in taking a trip on Amtrak, call their toll-free number (1-800-USA-RAIL) for information about accessibility of the stations and trains servicing the routes in which you are interested.

WHERE TO STAY

Many older hotels and most new ones in major U.S. cities now have rooms that have been especially adapted for guests with disabilities. With publication of the ANSI Standards for accessibility in 1976, concrete guidelines now exist for making hotel rooms, bathrooms, lobby areas, and meeting rooms accessible for disabled persons.[1]

When making travel plans, let the reservation person at the hotel know that you will require wheelchair accessibility. At that time, you also may wish to inquire about specific room arrangements and the layout of the bathroom. In some cases, different floor plans may be available so that you can choose a room that most closely meets your needs.

Several travel agencies specialize in making travel arrangements for clients with disabilities. Some of these agents are listed on pages 195 and 196. Since they regularly make arrangements for travelers with disabilities, they are a good source of information about airport accessibility, hotel suitability for disabled travelers, and other travel tips to make your trip more enjoyable.

WHERE TO EAT

Most of the major travel guides to restaurants now indicate whether or not the restaurants are wheelchair-accessible, in addition to providing information about cuisine, prices, atmosphere, and location. Other good sources of information are the travel agencies mentioned earlier and other individuals with disabilities. When checking a restaurant for accessibility, make sure to check the bathrooms as well as the seating and entrance areas. Many restaurants that appear to be "accessible" do not have accessible restrooms.

WHERE TO GO

You literally can go almost anywhere in a wheelchair that you could before you were injured. Do you want to go to a

---

[1] *American National Standard: Specifications for Making Buildings and Facilities Accessible to and Usable by Physically Handicapped People*, ANSIA A117.1-1980. New York: American National Standards Institute, Inc., 1980.

ball game? Most stadiums have special seating areas for wheelchair users and their companions. Would you like to go to Disney World or Busch Gardens? Most amusement parks have made as many of their facilities as possible accessible to users of wheelchairs and other visitors with disabilities. Accessible rides, concessions, eating facilities, and restrooms usually are marked clearly on maps distributed to visitors. Outdoor recreation areas, particularly those run by the federal government, often have facilities that have been adapted for people with disabilities, as have national monuments and museums. For further information on accessibility of specific areas of the country, see the resources listed at the end of this chapter.

LOCAL TRANSPORTATION

Until the late 1970s most public transportation systems such as buses and subways were completely inaccessible. Due primarily to intensive advocacy efforts of disability rights organizations, that picture is changing. Many major cities, including New York, Washington, D.C., Portland, Oregon, Denver, and Seattle have purchased accessible buses and have incorporated these buses into their regular schedule so that all potential riders can use the public transportation system. Some of these systems have combined this approach with the use of paratransit vehicles—taxis, dial-a-ride services, or van pools—to provide service in areas not served by accessible buses. In addition, mass transit systems such as the Bay Area Rapid Transit (BART) in San Francisco and metropolitan Washington, D.C.'s Metro have been designed to be accessible.

Local advocacy groups working in conjunction with city and county governments often are the instigators behind the development of accessible transportation systems. Consequently, the most up-to-date information about the accessibility of public transportation in your area can be obtained from local disability organizations and the local government's office for disabled individuals. The Paralyzed Veterans of America's national governmental affairs program also can provide you with information about transportation systems in your area and in other areas of the country that you may be visiting.

If your hometown does not have an accessible transportation system, you may wish to become an advocate yourself for more accessibility. Again, PVA can assist you by providing information on accessible transportation and negotiating techniques to use when discussing the problems with local decision makers.

Travel and transportation for persons with disabilities are much easier today than they were even 10 years ago. In many parts of the country, transportation officials and business owners have become aware of the importance of making their facilities accessible to disabled travelers and customers. This has come about because of a concerted effort on the part of disability rights advocates, lawmakers who recognized that people were being denied access to services that their tax dollars helped to support, and the cooperation of concerned business people. It now is possible for a person with a disability to get around reasonably well in the public sector without encountering architectural barriers every step of the way.

However, it is important to remember that every once in a while those barriers will become evident—usually it seems, at a time and place that prove to be most inconvenient. The best protection against those kinds of barriers is to be prepared by getting all the facts ahead of time so that you can minimize surprises. It also is helpful to sensitize your family and friends to the kinds of barriers that may exist, so that when they are in charge of planning a trip or evening out, they don't make reservations at a restaurant that turns out to be inaccessible or book you into an inaccessible hotel room.

Travel to an unknown place can be one of the most exhilarating experiences in life. There is no reason to miss out on those kinds of adventures just because you use a wheelchair.

TRAVEL AGENCIES AND TOUR GROUPS SERVING THE WHEELCHAIR TRAVELER

Access/Abilities
P.O. Box 458
Mill Valley, CA 94942
(415) 388-3250

Addie's You and I Travel Service
621 SW Alder #530
Portland, OR 97205
(800) 342-5500
In Oregon: (800) 342-5504
  (503) 222-9373

Anglo California Travel Service
4250 Williams Road
San Jose, CA 95129
(408) 257-2257

Catholic Travel Office
4701 Willard Avenue
Chevy Chase, MD 20815
(301) 657-9762

Directions Unlimited Accessible
  Tours
344 Main Street
Mt. Kisco, NY 10549
(800) 533-5343/(914) 241-1700

Doral Travel
1692 Route 88 West
P.O. Box 545
Brick, NJ 08723
(201) 840-0084

Emmett Travel, Inc.
4949 SW Macadam Ave.
Portland, OR 97201
(503) 223-5190

Evergreen Wings on Wheels Tours
19505 (L) 44th Avenue West
Lynnwood, WA 98036-5699
(800) 562-9298
In Washington: (800) 435-2288
  (206) 776-1184

Firstworld Travel
193 Country Club Gate
Pacific Grove, CA 93950
(408) 373-8454

Flying Wheels Travel
143 West Bridge Street
Box 382
Owatonna, MN 55060
(800) 533-0363/(507) 451-5005

Happy Holiday Travel
2550 NE 15th Avenue
Wilton Manors
Fort Lauderdale, FL 33305
(305) 561-5602

Helping Hand Tours, Inc.
A Division of Potomac Tours, Inc.
1314 Pennsylvania Ave., S.E.
Washington, D.C. 20003
(202) 546-9494

Mobility Tours
26 Court Street
Brooklyn, NY 11242
(718) 858-6021/858-5404
TTY (718) 625-4744

Nautilus Tours
5435 Donna Avenue
Tarzana, CA 91356
(818) 343-6339

Reprinted with permission from *Paraplegia News*, April, 1986.

New Haven Travel Service
900 Chapel St., Suite 325
New Haven, CT 06510
(800) 243-1806
In Connecticut: 772-0060

People and Places, Inc.
320 Central Park Plaza
Buffalo, NY 14214
(716) 838-4444

Society for the Advancement of
  Travel for the Handicapped
  (SATH)
26 Court Street
Brooklyn, NY 11242
(718) 858-5483

Travel Helpers Ltd.
160 Duncan Mill Road
Don Mills, Ontario
M3B 1Z5
Canada
(416) 443-0583

Travel Information Service
Moss Rehabilitation Hospital
Twelfth Street and Tabor Road
Philadelphia, PA 19141

Whole Person Tours, Inc.
P.O. Box 1084
Bayonne, NJ 07002-1084
(201) 858-3400 (call collect)

SUGGESTED READINGS

Access Chicago: A Guide to the City. Rehabilitation Institute of Chicago,
  345 E. Superior St., Chicago, IL 60611.
Accessibility. Minnesota Travel Information Center, Minnesota Office of
  Tourism, 240 Bremer Bldg., 419 N. Robert St., St. Paul, MN 55101.
Access New York City. Junior League of City of New York. Available
  through Eastern Paralyzed Veterans Association, 432 Park Avenue So.,
  New York, NY 10016.
Access Travel, A Guide to Accessibility of Airport Terminals. Architectural
  and Transportation Barrier Compliance Board, 330 C St., Room 1010,
  Washington, DC 20202.
*Assessment of Low-Cost Elevators for Near Term Application in Transit
  Stations* (July 1982). U.S. Dept. of Transportation, Transportation Sys-
  tems Center, Cambridge, MA.
Barrier Free Surface Transportation Terminals: Design Considerations.
  Ball Berezowsky Associates, Montreal, Canada. Prepared for the
  Urban Transportation Research Board, Canadian Surface Transpor-
  tation Administration, Transport Canada, 1000 Sherbrooke St., W.,
  P.O. Box 549, Montreal, Quebec H3A 2R3 Canada.
Cannon, D., and Rainbow, F.: *Fixed-Route vs. Paratransit Transportation*.
  Available through Paralyzed Veterans of America, 801 Eighteenth St.,
  N.W., Washington, DC 20006.
Cannon, D., and Rainbow, F. (1980): *Full Mobility: Counting the Costs and
  Alternatives*. American Coalition of Citizens with Disabilities, Wash-
  ington, DC.
Cannon, D., and Rainbow, F.: *Legislative Background on Transportation*

Access. Available though Paralyzed Veterans of America, 801 Eighteenth St., N.W., Washington, DC 20006.

Casey, R. F. (1981): *The Accessible Fixed-Route Bus Service Experience.* U.S. Department of Transportation Research and Special Programs Administration, Transportation Systems Center, Cambridge, MA.

Comments on Transportation for Handicapped Persons (June 1980). U.S. Dept. of Transportation, Washington, DC.

Denver Busing Its Disabled (Summer 1983). Accent on Living, Bloomington, IL.

Escalator Modification for the Handicapped (July 1980—Phase I Final Report). U.S. Dept. of Transportation, Urban Mass Transportation Administration, Washington, DC.

An Evaluation of Making Rail Transit Accessible to Handicapped Persons, A National Summary of Cost Estimates (April 1980). Transportation System Center. Prepared for the U.S. Department of Transportation, Urban Mass Transportation Administration, Washington, DC.

Evaluation Report on Five Wheelchair Life Options for Installation in Transit Coaches (January 1979). Metro Transit Staff, Seattle, WA.

The Handicapped Driver's Mobility Guide (1981, 3rd ed.). American Automobile Association, Falls Church, VA.

The Handicapped Traveller: A Guide for Travel Counsellors. Canadian Institute of Travel Counselors, 2333 Dundas Street, West, Suite 302, Toronto, Ontario, Canada M6R 3A6.

Hecker, H.: *Travel for the Disabled.* Twin Peaks Press, Box 8097, Portland, OR 97207.

International Directory of Access Guides (1981/1982). Rehabilitation International USA, Inc., 20 West 40th St., New York, NY 10018.

Jones, N. L. (April 1983): *Accessibility of Transportation for Disabled Persons: Legal Issues and Judicial Decisions.* Congressional Research Service, The Library of Congress, Washington, DC.

LTD Travel (quarterly newsletter). Order from LTD Travel, 116 Harbor Seal Court, San Mateo, CA 94404.

Mass transit (October 1981). *Paraplegia News,* 35(10).

Mass Transit. Mass Transit, 337 National Press Bldg., Washington, DC 20045.

McFarland, S. R. (June 1982): Personal Licensed Vehicles for Disabled Persons. *Paraplegia News* 36(6): 33–38.

Meier, H. (1981): *Accessible Public Transit Systems: A History and Overview of Accessible Transit Provisions in the United States.* United Cerebral Palsy Association, San Francisco, CA.

Metro. Bobit Publishing Co, 2500 Artesia Blvd., Redondo Beach, CA.

Moakley, T. (January 1984): Keeping track of mass transportation. *Paraplegia News* 38(1):23–53.

Murphy, M. J., Stark, N. T., and Cheatham, B. L. (1981): Transportation. In: *Beyond Paternalism: Local Governments and Rights of the Disabled.* International City Management Association, Washington, DC.

Passenger Transport. American Public Transit Association, 1225 Connecticut Avenue, N.W., Suite 200, Washington, DC 20036.

Person licensed vehicles. *Workshop Proceedings* (February 1983). National Institute for Handicapped Research, Washington, DC 20202.

Report (July/August 1983), Vol. 9, No. 4. National Center for a Barrier Free Environment. Available through Paralyzed Veterans of America, 801 Eighteenth St., N.W., Washington, DC 20006.

Station Platform Rail Car Threshold Gap Study (March 1982). U.S. Dept. of Transportation, Transportation Systems Center, Cambridge, MA.

Status of Special Efforts to Meet the Needs of the Elderly and Handicapped (April 1982). U.S. General Accounting Office, Washington, DC.

Subway Stations Modernization (February 1979). New York Dept. of City Planning, New York.

Technical Report of the National Survey of Transportation Handicapped People (September 1978). Grey Advertising, Inc. Dept. of Transportation, Urban Mass Transportation Administration, Washington, DC.

Transit Station Use by the Handicapped: Vertical Movement Technology (April 1980). U.S. Dept. of Transportation, Washington, DC.

Transportation for the Elderly and Handicapped: Programs and Problems 2 (October 1980). U.S. Dept. of Transportation, Washington, DC.

Urban Transportation for Handicapped Persons: Alternative Federal Approaches (November 1979). Congressional Budget Office. U.S. Government Printing Office, Washington, DC.

Wheelchair Lifts on Transit Buses (December 1982). U.S. Dept. of Transportation Systems Center, Cambridge, MA.

Wheelchair Restraint System Design for Multi-Modal Transportation (July 1979). Douglas Ball, Inc., Transport Canada, Montreal, Quebec, Canada.

Wheelchair Tie-Down/Passenger Seat Prototype Development (November 1978). Douglas Ball, Inc., Transport Canada Research and Development Center, Montreal, Quebec, Canada.

A World of Options: A Guide to International Educational Exchange, Community Service and Travel for Persons with Disabilities (1985–86). Mobility Intl. USA, P.O. Box 3551, Eugene, OR 97403.

CHAPTER 15

Minimizing the Damage After SCI

Lynn Phillips

The ultimate solution to the problem of spinal cord injuries is nothing short of full recovery of function and sensation. Until an effective treatment is found, however, many scientists and clinicians are focusing on several related areas of research. In this chapter, we will look at research geared toward minimizing the damage that occurs after a spinal cord injury. The next chapter will look at efforts to maximize the amount of function that is left. The final chapter will explore research that is looking at how the central nervous system responds to injury, how damage develops, and possible approaches toward increasing the amount of spinal cord regeneration.

THE NERVOUS SYSTEM

The spinal cord, eyes, and brain comprise the *central nervous system,* with all other nerves in the body belonging to the *peripheral nervous system.* The central nervous system serves as the central information-processing center for the entire body, sending messages to and from various parts of the body such as the heart, lungs, stomach, legs, arms, and fingers, and through the spinal cord to the brain and back, all within milliseconds. The conduit used to get this information to and from the central nervous system is the peripheral ner-

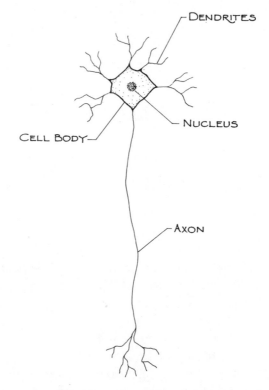

FIG. 15.1. Typical nerve cell.

vous system, which connects the central nervous system to the body's other organs.

It is estimated that there are more than 50 billion nerve cells in the human nervous system. Each nerve cell, or *neuron,* is composed of several distinct parts. The cell body or *soma* is that part of the cell which contains the *nucleus* (Fig. 15.1), and is usually smaller than two-thousandths of an inch. Many neurons also have at least one *axon,* whose primary function is sending out messages over considerable distances, often up to 2 to 3 feet. The primary purpose of *dendrites*—shorter versions of the axon, of which there can be many in a single neuron—is to receive messages from neighboring cells. Together, the dendrites and the cell axon comprise the nerve cell's *processes*. Each neuron, consisting of both its processes and cell body, can receive, transmit, and conduct messages from other cells.

The kinds of messages exchanged among different kinds of nerve cells are fundamentally very similar. However, these cells play many different roles in the human body. Some neurons, for example, are connected to muscles, whereas others exchange messages between the brain and the eye. The role of the nerve cell determines how many processes it will have, and how long its axons and dendrites will be. When one neuron transmits information to another, the site of that connection is called a *synapse*. Each neuron is involved in the establishment of a number of synapses, transmitting messages down its axon to a group of target cells, and receiving messages on its dendrites.

In addition to its information processing neurons, the nervous system contains a number of supporting cells called *glia*. Glial cells are even more plentiful than neurons; many of their functions are poorly understood, but they appear to assist neurons rather than to transmit nerve impulses. There are several different types of glial cells, all with unique and important functions. *Astrocytes,* for example, help to form scar tissue in response to injury to the central nervous system. They may also serve as a supporting structure for neurons and as a protective shield for synapses or groups of synapses. *Oligodendrocytes* are neuroglial cells which form *myelin*. Myelin forms the sheath of electrical insulation that covers the thicker axons in the CNS, and speeds electrical conduction in important pathways. *Microglial cells* are small cells that begin to reproduce rapidly after an injury to surrounding CNS tissue and then congregate in that area. *Ependyma,* another group of neuroglial cells, line the central canal of the spinal cord. Glial cells also isolate the CNS from blood-borne components, protecting sensitive neurons from toxic effects of many circulating substances that are harmless to other types of cells.

THE SPINAL CORD

The cells in which we have the greatest interest are those cells of the central nervous system, and particularly those cells which make up the spinal cord. All the cell types described above are present in the spinal cord. Like the rest of the brain, the spinal cord is composed of two major sections, *white matter* and *gray matter*. White matter is so named largely because of its high concentration of myelin, and is found around the periphery of the spinal cord. It contains glial cells as well as millions of axons that connect other cells in the body to neurons in the brain, or connect different functional regions of the central nervous system. The gray matter is shaped somewhat like an H or a butterfly in cross section and contains virtually all the neuronal cell bodies and synapses, along with many of their processes (Fig. 15.2).

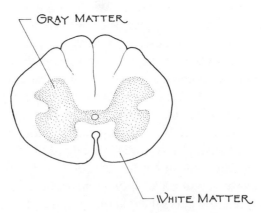

FIG. 15.2. Cross section of spinal cord.

RESPONSE TO INJURY

When a spinal cord injury occurs, the closely knit, intricate environment of neurons, their interwoven processes, and the glial cells in the space between the neurons become grossly disrupted. Axons that once established connections between a nerve cell body and other cells are cut or crushed and will no longer conduct nerve impulses. Consequently, the intercellular connections, or the *synapses,* no longer transmit information. The immediate damage in a spinal cord injury is thus due to the severing of electrical connections between brain and body (much like cutting a transatlantic cable), due to localized damage to axons at the site of the injury. This means that even the many undamaged cells elsewhere in the CNS can no longer communicate.

A traumatic spinal cord injury also initiates a series of secondary events that eventually enlarges the region of primary (and essentially nonrepairable) cell damage, and may result from abortive attempts by the body at self-repair. As in the primary injuries, by far the greatest deficit to the individual results from the interruption of *axons*—the part of the neuron that carries information to other cells, traveling in vast numbers through the spinal cord.

While many nerve pathways become dysfunctional immediately upon injury causing much paralysis and loss of sensation below the region of damage, the relevant cell bodies above and below the site of the injury are usually not killed and are capable of regenerating new axons and reestablishing synapses with their target cells. In some cases, such as damaged peripheral nerves, this regenerative process can lead to an almost complete restoration of function. This is also true for the CNS in our evolutionary ancestors, such as reptiles and amphibians. However, in mammals this natural regenerative process becomes disorganized by the consequences of local damage in the spinal cord. It is generally assumed that the glial ''scar'' that forms at the site of damage somehow prevents regeneration. Undoing this self-inflicted damage is thus the main hope for victims of CNS injuries, and an important focus for medical research.

WHY SPINAL CORD DAMAGE OCCURS

Immediately after injury, it appears that three major events occur that lead to cell death. These include damage to cell membranes; disruption of blood vessels that deprives nerve cells of oxygen and exposes them to toxic substances and the release of endorphins (and perhaps other toxic substances) into the blood.

The initial membrane damage that occurs immediately during and after injury appears to cause changes in the chemical composition of nerve cells, including increased calcium entry. This increased calcium level is toxic and causes degeneration and further damage to the cell. The ultimate result of these processes is localized cell death or *necrosis* near the site of injury.

Another immediate result of injury to the spinal cord is a local disruption of blood vessels. In the hours and days following injury, this disruption in the blood supply prevents nutrients and oxygen from reaching the nearby tissues, exposes neurons to toxic blood substances, and causes swelling or *edema* which further compresses these surrounding cells, leading to additional neuronal death.

Endorphins are natural pain-relieving proteins found in the human body. When a traumatic injury occurs, endorphins are released, presumably to counteract the pain that results. It is believed that these endorphins have a negative effect in the case of spinal cord injury, reducing blood flow to the injured area along with pain. This decreased blood flow could starve nerve cells of oxygen and other essential nutrients, causing further cell death.

APPROACHES TO MINIMIZING DAMAGE

Once traumatic injury has occurred, little can be done to stop or reverse the immediate effects of the primary lesion such as the initial damage to cell membranes and disruption of blood flow. However, clinicians and researchers have theorized that the extent of the ultimate damage that occurs to the spinal cord could be minimized if the sequence of destructive reactions within the spinal cord could be interrupted. Thus an important goal for much of the research in laboratories and clinics throughout the world is an effort to minimize the secondary damage that occurs as a result of a traumatic insult to the spinal cord. Investigators have suggested a variety of experimental treatment methods for both laboratory and clinical use. The value of these methods has sometimes been debunked, as the hypotheses upon which their usefulness might be based turned out to be incorrect. Others have failed to gain acceptance because controlled trials have yielded inconclusive results. Still others remain the subject of debate and speculation because adequate laboratory and/or clinical data have yet to be obtained.

CALCIUM CHANNEL BLOCKERS

One of the theories about the delayed effects of spinal cord injury is that the calcium levels in the spaces between cells decrease rapidly after injury and that calcium levels within the cells increase, a severe chemical imbalance that leads to cell death. Several investigators have thus proposed using calcium channel blockers in conjunction with high doses of corticosteroids or naloxone.[1] The purpose of using calcium channel

---

[1] A. I. Faden (1985): Pharmacologic therapy in acute spinal cord injury: Experimental strategies and future directions. In: *Central Nervous System Trauma Status Report*, edited by D. P. Becker and J. T. Povlishock, pp. 481–485. National Institute of Neurological and Communicative Disorders and Stroke, NIH, Bethesda.

blockers would be to prevent the movement of calcium from extracellular spaces into the cells, thus helping to maintain a more normal balance of this substance. To date, no definitive research results have been presented to indicate that calcium channels are involved in this damage, or that these channel blockers, either by themselves or in combination with other drugs, actually can inhibit secondary damage to the spinal cord after injury. However, this is one research approach that is still being tested.

CLONIDINE

Another possible source of damage results from the disruption of blood flow at the site of injury, denying nerve cells oxygen and other nutrients and exposing neurons to toxic blood substances. Clonidine, a drug now used to treat hypertension, or high blood pressure, was thus proposed in the 1970s and early 1980s as a possible treatment for acute spinal cord injury. Theoretically, clonidine was supposed to help maintain near-normal blood pressure levels in individuals after injury, limiting edema or swelling at the site of the lesion so that blood flow could be maintained to prevent further cell damage. In one report, which was published in a respected scientific journal, an investigator claimed that he had restored walking in paralyzed cats, and that function improved in 30 humans who were given the drug, although none was able to walk again. However, other investigators have been unable to reproduce the results, and serious objections were raised to the research protocol employed. Consequently, it would appear at this time that clonidine has little merit as a possible treatment for spinal cord injury.

DIMETHYL SULFOXIDE

Dimethyl sulfoxide (DMSO) is an industrial solvent that in recent years has been suggested to have several clinical applications, including the ability to limit spinal cord damage after a traumatic injury. It has two properties in particular that were seen as potentially helpful for application to SCI. First, it reduces swelling, or edema. Second, it can be absorbed through the skin easily, and would thus be a potentially non-invasive method of treatment. Investigators who have used DMSO in experimental situations also suggest that DMSO may help to stimulate blood flow through the injured area, maintaining the supply of oxygen to injured neural tissue.[2]

Several teams of respected investigators have conducted research on DMSO, and one reported positive results in a study of dogs.[1]

However, these results have not yet been replicated by others, so that potential benefit of DMSO as an aid to functional recovery after spinal cord injury is still very much in doubt.

ENZYME THERAPIES

A treatment technique which generated a lot of attention in the popular press was the reported use of "enzyme therapy" in the Soviet Union. Researchers in Leningrad claimed that by injecting enzymes into the spinal cord or into the bloodstream they were able to increase function in injured animals. In addition, they claimed that these enzyme injections helped to reduce mortality and infection, reduced scar formation and cavitation at the site of the lesion, and promoted the development of new blood vessels in the injured area. These claims were important because the formation of scar tissue appears to be a major reason for the fact that injured nerve cells are unable to reestablish connections with their target cells. The Leningrad group also claimed to have begun human clinical trials of the enzyme therapy.

When news of their work reached this country the Russian

---

[2] J. C. de la Torre (1981): *Spinal Cord Injury: Review of Basic and Applied Research,* unpublished data.

researchers were invited to the United States to present their results, and several American physicians went to the Soviet Union to observe what was occurring there. It soon became evident that the Soviets had made an important error in their research protocol, and that none of their human subjects were actually recovering any function beyond what could be expected from the intensive physical therapy and rehabilitation program which the Soviets were providing in addition to the enzyme therapy.

Unfortunately, several Americans spent large amounts of money to go to Leningrad, and participated in a program that ultimately provided no more relief for their trauma than they could have received with conventional therapy in the United States. The entire episode also raised false hope for many spinal cord–injured Americans, who felt that if only they had the money to go to the Soviet Union they would be "cured."

FREE RADICAL SCAVENGERS

One of the possible consequences of ischemia (the decreased blood flow that occurs in the injured area) is that molecules with unpaired electrons might be released, and that these highly reactive "free radicals" would then chemically attack other substances. This could cause chemical damage to otherwise uninjured parts of the CNS, leading to further cell death. Several research groups have proposed, therefore, to use antioxidants or *free radical scavengers* to block any attempt by such molecules to combine inappropriately with other molecules. Some of the suggested free radical scavengers include vitamins C and E, which are often combined with steroids.[1]

No value of these free radical scavengers in alleviating the secondary damage that occurs after spinal cord injury has yet been established. Nevertheless, the theories upon which their use was proposed may have some validity, and several research groups are continuing research in this area.

HYPERBARIC OXYGEN

Hyperbaric oxygen (HBO) is another therapy which has been recommended over the years for various uses. Its application to acute spinal cord injury has been proposed on the basis that exposure to high pressures (in a closed chamber) will facilitate oxygen delivery to the injured area, thus reducing the ischemic damage that occurs as a result of decreased blood flow. Hyperbaric oxygen may be of some use in cases of acute compression injuries, but it is not a widely accepted therapy at this point, and therefore is used rarely in the treatment of acute SCI.

HYPOTHERMIA

Hypothermia, or cooling of the injured spinal cord, has been proposed because cooling theoretically might help to reduce swelling around the injured area and thus prevent further cell death. Various methods of cooling the injured cord have been attempted in laboratory studies, but use of this approach has several inherent problems. First, for hypothermia to be used over a long period of time, the spinal cord must be exposed, and this involves additional risks to the patient. Second, no one yet has established practical guidelines for how long and at what temperature the cord should be cooled. Consequently, hypothermia remains a controversial, awkward, and as yet untested approach to acute SCI treatment.

NALOXONE

One of the theories about secondary spinal cord damage is that endorphins—the body's natural anesthetics—are released in the CNS after injury, where they further decrease blood flow to the injured area, in turn exacerbating the series of damaging events. Naloxone, an opiate antagonist, blocks the action of endorphins, and therefore may be effective in limiting further damage to the spinal cord. Initial animal studies with naloxone have shown positive results, and it is currently being tested in human clinical trials.

Naloxone appears to have several problems, however. First, by blocking the action of endorphins, naloxone also limits the body's ability to fight pain. Second, indications are that large doses of naloxone are required to be effective, but the use of high doses of such a potent drug in controlled clinical trials is unlikely to occur because of increased risks of toxic side effects. Consequently, controlled trials of naloxone are only being carried out using much smaller doses, a precaution which may lead only to inconclusive results. Nevertheless, naloxone is one drug which may eventually be helpful to newly injured individuals.

THYROTROPIN-RELEASING HORMONE

Thyrotropin-releasing hormone, or TRH, has many of the same properties as naloxone. It acts as an opiate antagonist and therefore assists the body in maintaining blood flow to the injured area. Unlike naloxone, however, it does not block the pain-relieving properties of endorphins, so the body's mechanism for fighting pain is not affected. Successful laboratory trials of TRH have been reported, and other research groups are now attempting to reproduce those results. Clinical trials of TRH recently have been initiated as well, and the results of those trials could be forthcoming within the next few years.

CORTICOSTEROIDS

One of the most controversial treatments for acute SCI is the use of corticosteroids in an attempt to prevent secondary damage after injury. These steroids are known to have strong anti-inflammatory properties, which theoretically could make them useful in reducing swelling and localized tissue damage at the site of injury. They also reportedly are useful in keeping cells and blood vessels intact, and so may contribute to stabilizing the chemical balance of the spinal cord after injury.

Steroids have been used routinely in the treatment of other acute injuries for years, but since controlled clinical trials had not been done, their use was based more on belief in their effectiveness than on proof. In the 1970s, the National Institute of Neurological and Communicative Disorders and Stroke (NINCDS) sponsored a multicenter clinical trial of the steroid *methylprednisolone*. The results of the study were inconclusive, partly because the dosages used were not as high as those that proponents claimed were necessary for effectiveness.

Many clinicians who have used steroids routinely in the past have now discontinued this practice due to an increasing body of data indicating that steroids are not particularly helpful in the treating of acute SCI. However, it remains a highly controversial subject to this day.

SUMMARY

None of the treatment techniques for acute SCI that have been proposed address all of the secondary complications of traumatic injury. It is unlikely, therefore, that any single "miracle drug" or treatment will be able to stop completely the damage that occurs after injury. It also is important to realize that even the most promising of the treatments outlined in this chapter do not attempt to reverse damage that already has occurred as a result of injury; rather, their purpose is to limit further damage.

What appears most feasible is that a combination of therapeutic interventions may minimize secondary damage after injury. Such an integrated approach really cannot be tested adequately, however, until the efficacy and mechanisms of each individual treatment approach have been determined. Once those questions have been answered definitively, scientists will be able to look objectively for combination treatments that effectively minimize additional cell damage after injury.

SUGGESTED READINGS

Becker, D. P., and Povlishock, J. T. (eds.) (1985): Central Nervous System Trauma Status Report. National Institute of Neurological and Communicative Disorders and Stroke, National Institutes of Health, Bethesda, MD 20814.

Controversies in spinal cord research (December 1984). *Paraplegia News*, 38(12):15.

The NINCDS Today (1981). National Institute of Neurological and Communicative Disorders and Stroke, Bethesda, MD. NIH Publication No. 82-2100.

Spinal Cord Injury and Nervous System Trauma (1981). National Institute of Neurological and Communicative Disorders and Stroke, Bethesda, MD. NIH Publication No. 81-1617.

CHAPTER 16

The Challenge to Restore Function to Paralyzed Limbs

Howard Chizeck

Historically, there have been many people who offered hope and "cures" for spinal cord injuries using devices chemical, mechanical, electrical, and spiritual. Testimonials of cures abound, primarily because the terms "paraplegia" and "quadriplegia" loosely describe a number of different conditions. Many readers of this book may have partial control of their limbs and may retain some sensation in them; the spinal cord nerves connecting to those limbs may not have been completely destroyed. For some people physical therapy may restore the use of the injured limbs. For others, improvement may occur independently. Other individuals may have no sensation and voluntary control of paralyzed limbs. Yet, all these various conditions are described as paralysis.

In the last two decades, researchers have begun to stimulate paralyzed limbs electrically in an effort to restore function to paralyzed muscles. At least 12 research centers worldwide are investigating ways to apply, control, and coordinate such electrical stimulation, which is called functional neuromuscular stimulation (FNS). The results so far are promising: These experimental techniques have enabled a small, carefully se-

Reprinted with permission from *Technology Review,* M.I.T. Alumni Association © 1985.

lected group of individuals with paraplegia to walk hundreds of meters in the laboratory, using walkers for support. Some have walked tens of meters with crutches, which afford a greater measure of independence. An even smaller number have climbed up and down stairs equipped with two hand railings, or have negotiated common stairs having one hand railing and a crutch.

In other labs (and in the home), a small number of people with quadriplegia have attained enough control of their paralyzed hands and forearms to accomplish simple but important tasks, such as feeding themselves, combing their hair, and brushing their teeth. These achievements could mean the difference between total dependence on other people and some sense of self-sufficiency.

For both quadriplegics and paraplegics, devices that can restore function in paralyzed limbs promise a new and exciting measure of independence. However, it is important to realize that these devices are still experimental. A long list of difficult technical problems remains to be solved before such devices can leave the laboratory for widespread use. Unfortunately, that is not always the message that has been delivered to the public through recent articles and television shows. Such accounts may have raised false hopes in many people with spinal cord injuries and their families. Many investigators fear that these overblown media accounts will not only disappoint patients but impede future work in the field.

The truth is that no commercial FNS devices are now available that provide spinal cord–injured people with the ability to walk and negotiate stairs, or that enable quadriplegics to have hand and forearm control. Furthermore, such devices are not expected to be widely available in the near future.

The only commercial FNS devices now available are those that help correct relatively minor gait problems with foot drop that usually occur when a patient is recovering from a stroke and only the lower leg remains paralyzed. The person therefore has difficulty controlling the movement of that foot.

External bracing systems (of the hip, knee, ankle, and foot) with added electrical stimulation are becoming available. However it is not yet clear what kinds of people, if any, will use these devices for daily mobility. The past history with nonelectric orthotics is not encouraging.

Having said all this, I must note that current progress in this field is very promising. While major advances are not on the immediate horizon, the future of FNS devices is bright.

APPROXIMATING NATURE—CRUDELY

Before considering how these artificial devices work, it is useful to review once again how the original equipment works. In all vertebrate animals, motion is accomplished when muscles contract. The muscles are turned on electrically by signals carried by nerves, which form the wiring of the motor-control system. Some nerves run from the spinal cord to the muscles, carrying signals that trigger movement. Most of these signals originate in the brain. Other nerves carry sensory information from the muscles, joints, and skin to the spinal cord and ultimately to the brain.

Sometimes the sensory information received at the spinal cord is enough to trigger the nerves that control movement. For instance, if you step on a piece of glass, the resulting sensation of pain triggers the nerves to command your foot to lift. This is called a reflex action because the information does not need to reach the brain to elicit a response.

When your spinal cord is injured, motor-control signals from the brain to the muscles may be disconnected. As a result, you are unable to move certain muscles voluntarily. The higher the injury in the spinal cord, the more muscles will be paralyzed. While lower-level injury may result in paralysis of the legs, injury to the upper parts of the spinal cord may mean paralysis of the legs, trunk, and arms.

If your spinal cord is injured, the pathway for feeding sensory information to the brain may also be disconnected. As a result, you will have impaired (or no) sensation from the areas connected by nerves to the spinal cord below the injury level. However, reflexes will still exist.

The hope is to develop "neural prosthetic" devices that can at least partially replace the function of the injured spinal cord. The problem, however, is much more difficult than simply restoring signal transmission. Researchers must find some way of approximating the extraordinarily complex system for human motor control.

In this system, each single motor nerve cell (motor neuron) activates hundreds or thousands of muscle fibers. Fibers are the cells in muscles that, when activated by an electrical signal, essentially convert chemical energy that the body derives from food into contractive force. Each muscle fiber receives its stimulus from only one motor neuron. A motor and all of its associated muscle fibers are together called a *motor unit.*

For movements such as walking or grasping an object with one hand, the central nervous system coordinates all the sensory information coming in with motor commands going out to the many muscles involved in producing the desired movement. In a sense, the human nervous system is an extremely complicated parallel processor, receiving, coordinating, and transmitting an enormous number of signals simultaneously.

At this stage, researchers are not even attempting to reproduce this natural motor-control system in its full complexity. Instead, they are concentrating on developing substitute systems that can achieve rudimentary motor control over paralyzed limbs.

HISTORY OF ELECTRICAL STIMULATION

The use of electrical stimulation for medical purposes has a long and somewhat dubious history. As early as 46 A.D., the Roman physician Scribonius Largus prescribed the use of the torpedo fish, an electric ray fish, to treat headaches and gout.

The torpedo fish was to be placed over the painful spot, where it would deliver a numbing electrical shock.

Then, in the 1740s, when scientists first learned to produce electricity and store it in a Leyden jar, electrical cures where reported for paralysis, kidney stones, epilepsy, and heart pain, as well as other ailments. Among the early practitioners of electrical stimulation was Benjamin Franklin, who used an electrostatic generator with Leyden-jar storage to treat patients suffering from convulsions, reportedly with good results.

The first use of electrical stimulation to contract muscles is commonly attributed to Luigi Galvani in 1791. Galvani produced the contractions by conducting electricity from a metal rod through the nerve and muscle of a frog's leg to another metal rod. Alessandro Volta verified Galvani's experimental results and corrected his idea that the source of electricity was the animal rather than the metal rods.

The modern use of electrical stimulation to activate paralyzed muscles is at least 25 years old. In 1960, Adrian Kantrowitz enabled a man with paraplegia to stand for several minutes by stimulating the muscles in his legs. The current, when switched on, created an electric field between a "ground" electrode and the active electrodes attached to the patient's skin. The electric field stimulated certain nerves in the patient's posterior that in turn caused muscles in the body to contract. The concentration straightened the patient's knees, allowing him to support his own weight. More recently, researchers have also developed techniques to deliver electrical stimulation through electrodes implanted in the target muscle, or surgically implanted around or on top of the actual nerves.

In 1970, researchers at the Rancho Los Amigos Hospital in California, and another group in Ljubljana, Yugoslavia, were the first to report standing and some forward motion in paraplegics. The Yugoslavian group used surface electrodes for stimulation, and has since enabled 27 patients to stand and 3 patients to walk using a walker or crutches.

In 1973, a person with paraplegia at the University of Virginia at Charlottesville walked approximately 40 feet using a walker for support. Stimulation was provided by a system of implanted electrodes. In 1983, Dr. Herwig Thoma of the University of Vienna also used implanted electrodes to enable two patients to stand and walk up to 100 meters with crutches. Several other laboratories, including the Pritzker Institute in Chicago, are working on FNS standing and walking systems as well.

Researchers working on these systems face a number of technological problems. For instance, while surface electrodes are the easiest to install since they remain outside the body, they are not very selective in the muscles they activate. That's because they must send their signals through the skin and fatty tissue, so they end up activating a number of different muscles and nerves. Furthermore, most surface electrodes must be replaced daily.

Electrodes that have been inserted into the muscle (*intramuscular electrodes*), which contain insulated stainless steel wires inserted through the skin into the muscle with deinsulated tips, are far more selective and reliable. They usually stimulate only the particular muscle (and nerves) into which they have been inserted. However, even though intramuscular electrodes do not require surgery, they are difficult to install. Electrodes surgically implanted around or on top of specific nerves may turn out to be the best for long-term use. However, because they are installed through surgery, they are not used for the temporary and often changing demands of research. The use of percutaneous intramuscular electrodes has primarily been carried out at Case Western Reserve University in Cleveland; it is now also being used at several other labs—most notably in Matsumoto, Sapporo, and Osaka in Japan.

The size of the electrodes and the materials they consist of present further technological limitations. Smaller electrodes made of materials more like human tissue must be developed before large numbers of electrodes can be implanted inside the body. Even more constraining is scientists' lack of in-depth knowledge about the basic biomechanical workings of the human body. We simply don't yet know how to coordinate the transmission of signals to and from a large number of elec-trodes simultaneously. No more than 50 electrodes are now being used even in the most sophisticated experimental sys-tems. The body's natural system of motor control, in contrast, employs thousands of simultaneous signals to regulate move-ment. Thus, today's artificial motor signals can command only large groups of motor units instead of individual units.

STIMULATING MUSCLES BY TRIAL AND ERROR

All existing neural prostheses work in similar ways (Fig. 16.1). First, the user generates commands either by making a physical movement or by turning a switch off or on. In some experimental systems, quadriplegics move their shoulder a certain way and a transducer mounted on the shoulder trans-lates that movement into an electrical signal. This signal then prompts muscles in the hand to contract. If the person pulls his or her shoulder back, for instance, the finger and thumb open and extend. In this way, a sequence of different shoulder movements can enable a person with quadriplegia to grasp and pick up a coffee cup.

In most experimental systems for paraplegics, the individual generates binary (on-off) signals using simple hand switches. The signals are sent to an electronic "stimulator," which uses this information to generate one electrical signal for each elec-trode. The electrodes carry these signals into the body, where they stimulate specific muscles. These muscles might control the way a particular joint should move, or how quickly the person's foot should be lifted off the floor. When all these muscles are stimulated in the proper sequence, acts such as

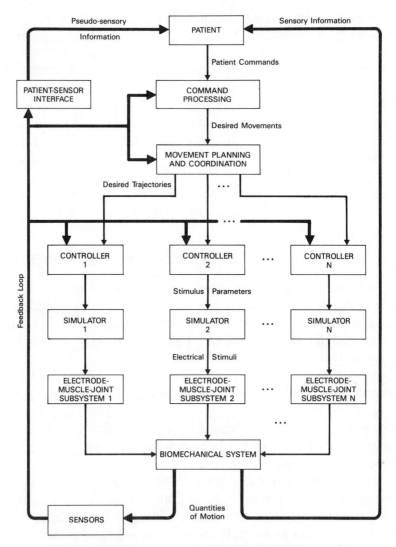

FIG. 16.1. General structure of neuroprosthetic system.

walking or grasping an object—which so many of us take for granted—can be achieved.

Researchers now use painstaking trial and error to determine the correct sequence of complicated movements needed for walking. These movements, which are different for every person, can also be determined mathematically from knowledge of the biomechanical system. However, this approach is again constrained by our limited knowledge of the body's biomechanics. Once scientists establish the movement sequence, they must determine the series of electrical stimuli needed to produce that movement and store it in the computer, to be refined as the individual learns to make the desired movement.

In most of these systems, the electrical stimulator is driven by a nonportable minicomputer, but work is progressing on more portable units. One of the stimulators used for walking at Case Western Reserve can be mounted on the individual's belt. The battery-powered device has a sophisticated microprocessor programmed with a stimulation sequence custom-made for each person who uses the system. The user communicates with this device via a finger-mounted ring-like switch.

This year some researchers have enabled paraplegics to walk much longer distances than ever before using more sophisticated control sequences. Under the direction of Byron Marsolais and colleagues at Case Western Reserve University, several research subjects at the Cleveland Veterans Administration Medical Center have been able to repeatedly move more than 400 feet using a rolling walker between rest stops, with maximum distances of about 1,000 feet. Several of these individuals can also repeatedly ascend and descend stairs having two handrails, and two of them are able to go up and down standard flights of single-rail stairs, using a quad crutch (a crutch with four supports at its base).

In all these experimental systems, some method of support is needed to sustain the person's weight and help maintain balance while he or she attempts to walk. The additional support can be provided by support harnesses, parallel bars, four-post walkers, rolling walkers, or crutches.

FINE-TUNING THE CONTROLS

A complicated sequence of signals must also be devised to restore function in the paralyzed hand muscles of people with quadriplegia. P. Hunter Peckham and his colleagues at Case Western Reserve have developed a system that relies on subtle shoulder movements to direct basic grasping movements in the hand. More than 10 research subjects have learned to use this system for such tasks as eating, typing (with a mechanical aid for pushing the keys), writing, drinking from rigid cups, and holding cigarettes. They can accomplish these tasks without the assistance of another person. The use of electrical stimulation coupled with tendon transfer surgery is also being studied by this group.

At present, most neural prostheses for paraplegics and quadriplegics rely on "open-loop control." The devices stimulate muscles based only on the user's commands and information previously stored in the computer. The controlling computer does not use measurements of movement to determine the stimulation signals.

In another more sophisticated strategy, sensors taped or strapped onto the person's limbs measure each limb's position and movements, and the computer uses this information to direct the stimulation of different muscles as needed. My colleagues and I at Case Western Reserve and the Cleveland VA Medical Center have developed such a system of "closed-loop control" in which four sensors measure the changing angle of the knees and ankles as our patients are standing (Fig. 16.2). We have found that the system helps people maintain their balance and perform other tasks without having to worry about whether their legs are about to buckle. Recent work has focused on reducing the amount of stimulation needed to maintain standing. In addition, closed-loop controllers that

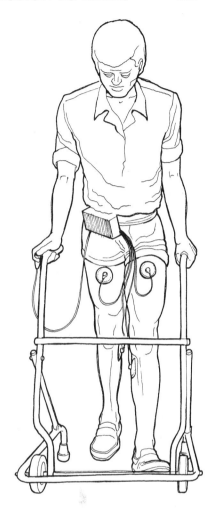

FIG. 16.2. Lower extremity FNS system being developed by researchers.

maintain hip position through the simultaneous stimulation of opposing muscles are currently being tested. Good control of hip and trunk position is essential for people with paraplegia to be able to perform functional tasks while standing.

A research team at Wright State University has also reported using closed-loop control strategies for walking as well as for standing—work that has been well-publicized in the popular media. More recently the group at Wright State has reported a change of direction, to the use of external orthotic braces augmented with electrical stimulation. Closed-loop control of the ankle during standing is also being investigated by researchers at the Pritzker Institute in Chicago.

A system of closed-loop control does offer enormous potential for helping people with spinal cord injury walk. Externally mounted sensors could be used to provide feedback from muscle movements as they happen and to time the next cycle of movements. For instance, information indicating that the right foot has reached the ground and is supporting weight might be used to initiate the next step with the left foot. Sensors may also eventually be used to measure and modify quan-

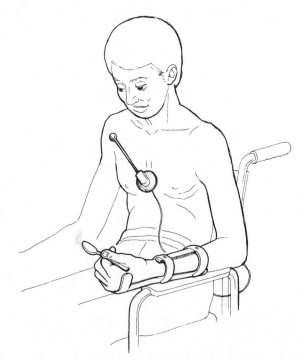

FIG. 16.3. Upper extremity FNS system.

tities of motion, such as the degree of force applied when the foot contacts the floor.

Several labs are also developing sensors to help quadriplegics regulate their hand motions when attempting to grasp a fork or coffee cup (Fig. 16.3). However, no one has yet developed an effective closed-loop control system for accomplishing either walking or grasping an object. The problem is once again technological: External sensors are difficult to calibrate and to attach in a fixed position. These drawbacks could be dangerous if the error produces a misstep when the person isn't ready to move. In addition, many people find such visible electronic gadgetry unsightly. Developing suitable sensors is a major technical challenge in producing effective FNS systems for both paraplegics and quadriplegics.

WHO WILL USE THEM AND WHO WILL PAY?

Perfecting the devices now being studied in research laboratories for reliable and functionally useful clinical use will take years. Today technicians must regularly adjust the neural prostheses used for walking. The devices also require a marathonlike effort from the research subjects since their muscles are easily fatigued from the constant artificial stimulation.

Most of the technological problems with neural prostheses eventually will be overcome. By the time they are, I hope we will have answered an often-neglected question: Who will use these devices? This question really has two parts. Which people, if given the choice, will use the systems, and which ones will be given the choice?

Despite the existence of walking aids such as long leg braces, most individuals who are paralyzed in both legs choose to use wheelchairs as their primary vehicle for mobility. This is simply because the physical effort associated with using braces does not justify the amount of increased access they afford. If you have paraplegia, you probably will use FNS systems only if they are relatively easy to wear and take care of, and if they do not make excessive demands on your energy and time. How these prostheses look is also important; many people don't wish to wear a device that attracts unwanted attention.

Most importantly, neural prostheses must provide you with capabilities you don't now have. Such systems must provide you with the ability not only to walk reasonable distances but also to overcome barriers such as stairs. Devices that help you stand must allow you to do so while engaged in significant, mind-consuming tasks. If the new devices don't provide these added capabilities, it is unlikely that you will abandon your wheelchairs because the costs associated with using the technology simply would not be worth the effort.

If you are a quadriplegic, however, the acceptance of a device that could help you use your hands may be a very different story. The ability to manipulate objects could mean the difference between dependence on attendant care and the ability to take control of many of your basic needs. There is also a strong financial reason for developing easy-to-use neural prostheses for people who are quadriplegic. Such devices theoretically could save millions of dollars in health care costs by reducing the need for attendant care and by increasing opportunities to develop skills that could lead to employment.

Although it is impossible to estimate accurately the eventual cost of these devices, they will probably be at least as expensive as an automobile. Even so, given the strong financial incentives, public and private health insurance companies may choose to cover such devices, making them affordable to most people with quadriplegia.

The balance of costs and benefits may be less compelling for devices that aid people with paraplegia. Insurance companies might argue that paraplegics can already get around with wheelchairs, and many have jobs. The intangible improvements to individuals' quality of life are not always the overriding concern of health care insurers. And with the growing push to contain medical costs, policymakers may decide that public health care programs such as Medicaid and Medicare cannot afford to pay for these devices. Thus, when they finally become commercially available, not all people who need them may be able to afford them.

The future of efforts to restore muscle function to disabled individuals through the use of electrical stimulation is promising. However, multidisciplinary teams of scientists, engineers, and health care professionals will have to work long and hard to solve difficult technical problems before these devices become widely available. This research should not be pressured by premature and exaggerated accounts of success in the popular press, which may raise false hopes among people with spinal cord injuries and damage the credibility of investigators in the field.

SUGGESTED READINGS

Barker, A. (December 1984): Functional electrical stimulation—current research yields hope for future. *Paraplegia News*.

Chizeck, H. J. (July 1985): Helping paraplegics walk: looking beyond the media blitz. *Technology Review*.

Maximizing function after spinal cord injury (December 1985). *Paraplegia News*. 39(12)23–39.

CHAPTER 17

The Search for a Cure

Lynn Phillips

The search to find a "cure" for spinal cord injury is a complex effort. One part of that search is to determine why the human CNS does not repair itself. That large question is comprised of a number of smaller, yet still complex, questions about the central nervous system. We know that lower animal species, such as reptiles and amphibians, have central nervous systems that can regenerate but that mammals do not. What do those less sophisticated animals have that our human system is lacking? We also know that the peripheral nervous system in humans can in principle repair itself. If you cut your finger and damage some nerves, for example, those nerves tend to reestablish their connections and you will eventually regain feeling in your finger. Why can this part of our nervous system repair itself, while the much more important brain and spinal cord cannot?

Answers to the fundamental questions regarding human CNS regeneration, therefore, depend on knowing how the human CNS reacts when it is injured. We know that catastrophic functional disruption occurs, but what sequence of events at the cellular level causes such a permanent loss of function?

Once we determine *what* happens after a spinal cord injury, we also need to know *why* it reacts as it does, *how* the process of nerve regeneration is regulated, and whether we can encourage this regenerative process to obtain complete restoration of function.

These are all difficult questions, and the possible approaches to each are limited by the current level of scientific knowledge and technology. Consequently, scientists all over the world are looking at separate parts of this general question in an effort to learn as much as possible about neurons such as those in the spinal cord and their reaction to injury, with the ultimate goal of identifying possible ways to reestablish injured connections.

The lack of progress in developing a cure for spinal cord and other traumatic injuries to the central nervous system is thus a direct consequence of our ignorance about the biological mechanisms that control neural development and regeneration. In fact, we still know remarkably little about the way animals develop from a single fertilized egg cell to a complex organism, possibly the single greatest mystery in biology. In particular, there is only the most rudimentary information about the ways growing axons guide their growth to the precise target cells with which they must connect both to establish their appropriate function and to survive.

It is known, however, that damaged adult neurons retain their embryonic ability to find the "right" target cells, particularly in lower vertebrates such as reptiles and amphibians. One of the more promising avenues of research thus centers upon discovering the differences between higher and lower animals that have reduced our adult ability to "repair" neural damage.

The other area of particular promise concerns research into the molecular basis of neural growth. This kind of research attempts to identify the molecules that play the critical role of controlling nerve growth and the ultimate regeneration (or development) of new synaptic contacts. Since the fundamental mechanisms that control nerve growth and synapse formation appear to be very similar in humans and other vertebrates, this form of "basic research" usually studies nerve growth in animal systems, or in particularly simple "isolated" systems such as cell culture.

It is, in fact, the extraordinary simplicity of these latter systems that makes them useful in determining the fundamental mechanisms we need to understand. The overwhelming problem for any analytic discipline, such as science, is complexity itself, which limits the usefulness of our most powerful forms of modern technology. For this reason it is virtually impossible to carry out profound scientific experiments on so complex a system as a spinal cord–injured person, even if such experimentation could be justified on ethical grounds. The mechanisms that regulate nerve growth and synapse formation must instead be studied first in simple isolated preparations, to identify the kinds of biological processes that control these important events. Once these are known, it becomes feasible to look at more complex cases, such as experimental animals and humans, for the aberrant events that prevent functional regeneration.

At present, very little is known about the processes that regulate nerve growth and synapse formation. One hypothesis is that target cells release hormonal-like substances, sometimes called *trophic factors,* that attract and sustain growing nerves. *Nerve growth factor* is one substance that could play such a role but works only with a few kinds of nerve cells. Considerable effort is being expended to find similar substances that affect other kinds of nerves, including those in the spinal cord. These efforts have not met with considerable success, and there is still some doubt whether trophic factors are actually the main means of directing and supporting nerve growth in an animal (or human).

Much recent research is focusing upon another possibility, that nerve growth and synapse regeneration are controlled by nonhormonal molecules associated with the *extracellular matrix,* structural proteins that surround neuronal cells, and may in many cases be produced by glial cells. This idea is quite consistent with the problems of spinal cord injury, where glial scar tissue (an inappropriate form of extracellular matrix) seems to block or misdirect the path of regenerating nerve fibers. Another emerging area, related to the above, surrounds experiments which suggest that nerve growth and synapse development could ultimately be controlled by the chemical interactions that occur when cells "touch" one another, or their surrounding extracellular matrix. These contacts may function like hormones, to keep the regenerating nerve cell alive and control the direction in which it grows. When the nerve axon grows to the right place, where its "target cell" lives, it is able to form a new synapse and thus establish a functional link between the brain and an "affector" organ such as muscle or sensory cell. Once we know how these molecules work to direct nerve growth, it should become possible to identify how inappropriate molecules impede nerve regeneration, and perhaps remove them. Alternatively, if the problem is really the *absence* of supportive molecules, we may be able to replace them with synthetic substitutes, again allowing nerve regeneration.

CURRENT THEORIES

In addition to attempting to understand the fundamental mechanisms underlying cell growth in the central nervous system, some scientists are exploring methods of encouraging nerve cells to establish useful connections; in some systems nerve cells *do* establish useful connections with their target cells. Such systems include lower animal models, embryos of animals at all developmental levels, and nerve cell growth in the peripheral nervous system. By looking at nerve cell development and the interaction between cells in systems that do regenerate new synaptic contacts, scientists are attempting to learn more about nerve cell growth.

A different approach being taken by other scientists is to look at spinal cord injuries in species that do not regenerate and then attempt to establish nerve growth through the injured area. Some investigators, for example, have attempted to transplant embryonic nerve tissue into injured CNS tissue to replace lost nerve cells and promote axonal regeneration. Investigators in Sweden and elsewhere have had limited success in transplantation of embryonic tissue into brain tissue in laboratory studies, but similar studies in the spinal cord have not yet yielded particularly encouraging results. So far, successful CNS transplants have been achieved only in attempts to replace lost *neurosecretory* tissues with embryonic equivalents, and there is little evidence yet that similar procedures will allow regeneration of the lost electrical connections that would be essential for any functional repair of the spinal cord.

Other scientists are attempting to encourage regrowth of nerve fibers by altering the environment in which the injured cells operate. Since a traumatic injury causes a severe chemical and electrical imbalance in the injured area, some scientists are looking at ways to change that environment, using chemical substances or electrical currents to provide an environment more conducive to orderly cell growth.

It appears that the glial "scar" may play an important role in preventing axonal regeneration. Consequently, some groups are studying this problem of glial scar formation by looking at lower vertebrates and in some cases peripheral nerves, where substantial regeneration does occur. In the frog, for example, CNS neurons from the retina grow precisely back to their target cells and reestablish vision. Because of instances such as these, it is possible that promoting functional neural regeneration could be a relatively simple process, achieved by either preventing or removing the obstacle that blocks an otherwise reliable biological repair mechanism.

One phenomenon that occurs after injury is that injured axons often do attempt to regrow, but in unproductive directions. This *sprouting* is being studied to see whether axons can somehow be encouraged to regrow in useful directions.

Until the central problem—understanding what guides nerve growth to the correct target cells, either in embryonic development or during instances of successful regeneration in other animals—is addressed, it is unlikely that a cure for spinal cord injury will be found. Despite the advances that have been made in recent years, our understanding of basic CNS development and regeneration is still rudimentary and, if we don't know how and why the system performs the way it does, it is difficult to develop ways to fix it when it is injured.

FEDERAL AND PRIVATE SUPPORT OF SPINAL CORD RESEARCH

The most realistic approach to the issue of spinal cord regeneration is to acknowledge that the problem is incredibly complex, and that answers will not come quickly. However, progress is occurring at a rapid pace, and many scientists now acknowledge that eventually spinal cord regeneration may be possible.

Until the early 1970s, it generally was assumed that regeneration or regrowth of damaged nerve cells in the central nervous system was an impossible task. Since that time, neurosciences have moved ahead significantly so that spinal cord regeneration is a reasonable dream, even if not a probable one for the near future.

The federal government is the single largest supporter of research in the United States that could yield insights into why the central nervous system does not regenerate. Through basic science research, which looks at the fundamental mechanisms that determine how the body works, to applied clinical studies, which test new approaches for treating diseases or conditions, scientists and clinicians are attempting to learn more about how the body responds to spinal cord injury. Engineers and clinicians also are looking at better ways to apply technology to aid disabled persons. While most of these studies are performed in universities and hospitals throughout the United States, much of the financial support for this work still comes from the federal government.

NATIONAL INSTITUTES OF HEALTH

The country's largest and best-known source of funding for medical research is the National Institutes of Health (NIH), located in Bethesda, Maryland. One of the NIH institutes, the National Institute of Neurological and Communicative Disorders and Stroke (NINCDS), provides the largest source of funding in the United States for neurological research, including research aimed at finding a cure for spinal cord injury. Although some of the basic research being done on the structure and behavior of nerve cells is relevant to what goes on after a spinal cord injury, NINCDS also has a special division which is dedicated to funding research directly related to stroke and trauma, as well as a special division for research on neural prostheses, or functional neuromuscular stimulation.

Other institutes within NIH also fund research that is relevant to spinal cord injury. The National Institute of Diabetes and Digestive and Kidney Diseases, for example, provides funding for research on urological problems. Since most individuals with spinal cord injury have associated complications with bladder and kidney function, some of the research sponsored by this institute is applicable to persons with spinal cord injuries. The National Institute of Arthritis and Musculoskeletal and Skin Diseases also funds research relevant to spinal cord injury.

VETERANS ADMINISTRATION

The Veterans Administration (VA) is a surprisingly large supporter of medical research in the United States, including research related to spinal cord injury. Research in the Veterans Administration is under the supervision of the Department of Medicine and Surgery. All medical and basic science research is coordinated through the office of the Assistant

Chief Medical Director (ACMD) for Research and Development. Rehabilitation research, including the development of new devices for spinal cord–injured persons, is coordinated through the Deputy Assistant Chief Medical Director (DACMD) for Prosthetics.

All VA research programs sponsor work that is relevant to spinal cord injury, but two are of special importance. The first is the Office of Regeneration Research Programs (ORRP), which coordinates all regeneration research projects that are funded by the Veterans Administration. The ORRP was established in 1980 and is headquartered at the Portland, Oregon, VA Medical Center. ORRP sponsors conferences and symposia on regeneration research in addition to funding regeneration research projects, and has published books based upon papers presented at these meetings.

The second is the VA's Rehabilitation Research and Development Service (Rehab R&D), which sponsors research related to rehabilitation, including the development of assistive aids and devices. Spinal cord injury is one of three special research foci of the Rehab R&D office. The other too are prosthetics and sensory aids.

The Veterans Administration's offices of Medical Research, Health Services Research and Development, and Cooperative Studies also fund research related to spinal cord injury. Health Services Research and Development recently conducted a feasibility study to determine whether the VA could track causes of death among spinal cord–injured veterans. The purpose of such a study would be to determine whether spinal cord–injured persons are more susceptible to certain causes of death than the general population. The Cooperative Studies Service conducted a multicenter clinical trial of acetohydroxamic acid (AHA or LithoStat) in VA spinal cord injury centers during the early 1980s to determine whether this drug is effective in inhibiting the growth of infectious urinary stones.

NATIONAL INSTITUTE OF DISABILITY RESEARCH AND REHABILITATION (NIDRR)

The National Institute of Disability Research and Rehabilitation (formerly the National Institute of Handicapped Research) was established by an act of Congress in 1978 and officially began operations on July 2, 1979. NIDRR is located in the Department of Education and supports Research and Training Centers (R&T Centers), research fellowships, and investigator-initiated research projects.

CENTER SPECIALTIES

One of the major effects of grant support by NIH, the VA, NIDRR, and the Rehabilitation Services Administration (RSA) has been to establish centers that are reknowned for their excellence in particular areas of research or treatment. The University of Virginia, for example, is one of the best-known centers for wheelchair research in the United States. As one of NIDRR's rehabilitation engineering centers (REC), the University of Virginia has developed a team of engineers and clinicians who specialize in all areas of wheelchair prescription and design, and who have played an active role in the development of international and U.S. standards for wheelchairs.

The University of Wisconsin at Madison has developed a nationally recognized program in the area of communications and computer usage for disabled persons. Their work includes the development of technological aids for nonverbal disabled persons as well as the development of computer technologies for severely disabled people.

The Veterans Administration, through its Rehabilitation Research and Development Service, has established three Rehab R&D centers at VA medical centers in Palo Alto, California; Hines, Illinois; and Decatur, Georgia. Each of the VA centers receives core funds to support a minimum level of research activity and then is encouraged to seek additional funds through the VA merit review process, NIH, NIDRR, or private organizations.

The Veterans Administration's 21 spinal cord injury centers, while primarily treatment centers, also provide research opportunities in clinically oriented spinal cord research. Physicians and other staff members at the VA SCI centers are encouraged to apply for research funds from the VA and other sources. RSA Model Regional SCI Centers also conduct research related to spinal cord injury.

PRIVATE FUNDING OF SCI RESEARCH

Although the bulk of funding for spinal cord injury research comes from the federal government, private organizations and foundations also contribute funds in this area. The Paralyzed Veterans of America's Spinal Cord Research Foundation (SCRF) was established in 1976 and has provided an average of approximately $500,000 in research grants each year since then to investigators in fields related to spinal cord injury. These include investigators in the field of regeneration research as well as those who are doing clinical research and device development. From its inception in 1976 through fiscal year 1986, SCRF provided over $4 million in research grants.

The American Paralysis Association (APA) and the Stifel Paralysis Research Foundation together provide funding for cure-oriented research and for projects that attempt to maximize function after spinal cord injury. In addition to funding investigator-initiated research, APA and the Stifel Foundation have developed Project TARGET, which funds specific projects targeted by the two sponsoring organizations and panels of experts as among the more promising areas of spinal cord regeneration research.

The National Spinal Cord Injury Association (NSCIA) in the past has concentrated on regeneration research and on basic science projects that will lead to a greater understanding of how the central nervous system works. NSCIA has funded fellowships for promising young researchers, and they have since the 1970s cosponsored with the Society for Neuroscience a biannual conference on regeneration. NSCIA currently sponsors research in a variety of fields related to spinal cord injury.

The Spinal Cord Society funds spinal cord research, with emphasis on a cure and on maximizing function after spinal cord injury. The National Easter Seal Society funds disability-related research which, although not focused specifically on spinal cord injury, includes development of devices for use by persons with disabilities.

Small, private foundations and civic and religious organizations sponsor individual research projects, as well. Information on these kinds of foundations can be obtained by contacting The Foundation Center, 888 Seventh Avenue, New York, New York 10106.

It may appear that support of spinal cord injury research is fragmented and undirected, but the truth of the matter is that most of the funders of research keep informal tabs on what others are funding, and most researchers in the area are familiar with other researchers who are doing similar kinds of work. Furthermore, plentiful opportunities exist for researchers to confer on a formal and informal basis at frequently held conferences and symposia. Consequently, although the funding "system" for spinal cord research may seem somewhat confusing and unorganized, it is a system that works fairly well.

The biggest single problem voiced by researchers in all aspects of this field is that the amount of support available does not begin to cover the need. Since the early 1980s, researchers have seen established programs being cut back to barely subsistence levels and the number of new grants decreased. This kind of budget crunching now will be felt most strongly during upcoming years, since fewer new investigators will have been able to enter the field.

SUMMARY

Although a cure for spinal cord injury has not yet been found, work in the past 15 years has led to increasing optimism that someday a cure will be found. In addition, advances in other areas such as improved medical care, increasing opportunities for rehabilitation, and the development of sophisticated adaptive devices ensure that people with spinal cord injuries are afforded many more opportunities than they were even a few years ago. Combined with changing attitudes on the part of society as a whole, employers, and public service personnel, life with a spinal cord injury does not have to be any less satisfying than was life before you became disabled.

SUGGESTED READINGS

The challenge of research (December 1983). *Paraplegia News,* 37(12)21–40.

From 'Regeneration' to Prosthesis: Research on Spinal Cord Injury (April 1981). *JAMA,* 245(13):1293–1301.

Heimer, L. (1983): *The Human Brain and Spinal Cord: Functional Neuroanatomy and Dissection Guide.* Springer-Verlag, New York, NY.

New focus on spinal cord injury (March 1981). *JAMA,* 245(12):1201–1206.

Spinal Cord Injury: Hope Through Research (1981). National Institute of Neurological Diseases and Stroke, National Institutes of Health, Bethesda, MD 20814.

Spinal Cord Regeneration—Promising Frontiers in Research. Paralyzed Veterans of America, 801 Eighteenth St., N.W., Washington, DC 20006.

Windle, W. F. (1980): *The Spinal Cord and Its Reaction to Traumatic Injury.* Marcel Dekker, Inc., New York, NY 10016.

Appendix 1. Treatment Centers

RSA MODEL REGIONAL SPINAL CORD INJURY CENTERS

Spain Rehabilitation Center
University of Alabama in Birmingham
Birmingham, AL 35294
(202) 934-3450

Rancho Los Amigos Hospital
Harriman Bldg. 121
7601 E. Imperial Hwy.
Downey, CA 90242
(213) 922-7167

Craig Hospital
Rocky Mountain SCI Center
3425 Clarkson Street
Englewood, CO 80110
(303) 789-8000

The Shepherd Spinal Center
2020 Peachtree Road, NW
Atlanta, GA 30309
(404) 352-2020, Ext. 179

Northwestern University Medical
    Center
Northwestern Memorial Hospital
Suite 619
250 E. Chicago Avenue
Chicago, IL 60611
(312) 908-3425

Boston University
N.E. Regional SCI Center
75 E. Newton Street
Boston, MA 02118
(617) 638-7300

Rehabilitation Institute Inc.
SE Michigan SCI System
261 Mack Blvd.
Detroit, MI 48201
(313) 494-9731

University of Michigan
Physical Medicine and Rehabilitation
E32528 University Hospital
Box 33
Ann Arbor, MI 48109
(313) 764-9401

New York University Medical Center
Rusk Institute of Rehab Medicine
400 East 34th Street
New York, NY 10016
(212) 340-6125

Strong Memorial Hospital
University of Rochester Medical
    Center
601 Elmwood Avenue
Rochester, NY 14642
(716) 275-3271

Jefferson Medical College
Thomas Jefferson University
11th and Walnut Streets
Philadelphia, PA 19107
(215) 928-6573

The Institute for Rehabilitation and
Research
Texas Medical Center
1333 Moursund Avenue
Houston, TX 77030
(713) 797-5910

University of Virginia Medical Center
Box 159
Department of Orthopedics and
Rehabilitation
Charlottesville, VA 22908
(804) 924-8578

Program Coordinator:

Medical Sciences Program, NIDRR
Mary E. Switzer Bldg. MS 2305
303 "C" Street, S.W.
Washington, DC 20202
(202) 732-1194

NIDRR REHABILITATION ENGINEERING CENTERS

Center	Service
Rancho Los Amigos Hospital, Inc. Professional Staff Association 7413 Golondrinas Street Downey, CA 90242 (213) 922-7167	Functional electrical stimulation
Electronic Industries Foundation Suite 700 1901 Pennsylvania Avenue, N.W. Washington, DC 20006 (202) 955-5823	Industry and evaluation of technology
Northwestern University Regional Engineering Center 633 Clark Street Evanston, IL 60201 (312) 649-8560	Prosthetics and orthotics
Cerebral Palsy Research Foundation of Kansas, Inc. 2021 North Old Manor Wichita, KS 67208 (316) 588-1888	Work site modification

Center	Service
Louisiana Tech University Department of Biomedical Engineering P.O. Box 7923 T3 Rustin, LA 72172 (318) 257-4562	Personal licensed vehicles
Harvard—MIT Children's Hospital Medical Center 300 Longwood Avenue Boston, MA 02115 (617) 735-6594	Quantification of human performance

Tufts—New England Medical Center
Department of Rehabilitation
  Medicine
171 Harrison Avenue
Boston, MA 02111
(617) 956-5031/5625
	Research on nonvocal communication
	  systems

University of Minnesota
Department of Physical Medicine and
  Rehabilitation
c/o ORA
1919 University Avenue
St. Paul, MN 55455
(612) 373-8990
	Improved quantification of human
	  performance

Dallas Rehabilitation Foundation 7850 Brookline Road Dallas, TX 75235 (817) 273-2249	Quantification of human performance
Southwest Research Institute Electronic Systems Division P.O. Drawer 28510 6220 Culebra Road San Antonio, TX 78284 (512) 684-5111	Evaluation of technology

Center	Service
University of Virginia Medical Center Department of Orthopedics and Rehabilitation P.O. Box 159/UVA Charlottesville, VA 22908 (804) 977-6730	Wheelchair systems and specialized seating
University of Wisconsin Board of Regents 750 University Avenue Madison, WI 53706 (608) 262-6966	Access to communication, control, and information-processing systems

NIDRR INTERNATIONAL REHABILITATION ENGINEERING CENTER

Center	Service
Rehabilitation Institute University of Ljubljana Department of Physical Medicine and Rehabilitation Linhartova 51 61000 Ljubljana, Yugoslavia	Functional electrical stimulation

VETERANS ADMINISTRATION SPINAL CORD INJURY CENTERS

Chief, SCI Service
Veterans Administration Medical
  Center
5901 East Seventh Street
Long Beach, CA 90822
(213) 498-1313

Chief, SCI Service
Veterans Administration Medical
  Center
3801 Miranda Avenue
Palo Alto, CA 94304
(415) 493-5000

Chief, SCI Service
Veterans Administration Medical
  Center
(SCI Outpatient Clinic)
Sepulveda, CA 91343
(213) 891-7711

Chief, SCI Service
Veterans Administration Medical
  Center
1201 Northwest 16th Street
Miami, FL 33125
(305) 324-4455

Chief, SCI Service
Veterans Administration Medical
  Center
1400 Veterans of Foreign Wars
  Parkway
West Roxbury, MA 02132
(617) 583-4500

Chief, SCI Service
Veterans Administration Medical
  Center
St. Louis, MO 63125
(314) 487-0400

Chief, SCI Service
Veterans Administration Medical
  Center
East Orange, NJ 07019
(201) 676-1000

Chief, SCI Service
Veterans Administration Medical
  Center
130 Kingbridge Road
Bronx, NY 10468
(212) 584-9000

Chief, SCI Service
Veterans Administration Medical
  Center
13000 North 30th Street
Tampa, FL 33612
(813) 972-2000

Chief, SCI Service
Veterans Administration Medical
  Center
Augusta, GA 30910
(404) 724-5116

Chief, SCI Service
Veterans Administration Medical
  Center
Hines, IL 60141
(312) 343-7200

Chief, SCI Service
Veterans Administration Medical
  Center
940 Belmont Street
Brockton, MA 02401
(617) 583-4500

Chief, SCI Service
Veterans Administration Medical
  Center
Castle Point, NY 12511
(914) 831-2000

Chief, SCI Service
Veterans Administration Medical
  Center
10701 East Boulevard
Cleveland, OH 44106
(216) 791-3800

Chief, SCI Service
Veterans Administration Medical
  Center
San Juan, PR 00936
(809) 758-7575

Chief, SCI Service
Veterans Administration Medical
  Center
1030 Jefferson Avenue
Memphis, TN 38104
(901) 523-8990

Chief, SCI Service
Veterans Administration Medical
  Center
2002 Holcombe Blvd.
Houston, TX 77031
(713) 795-4411

Chief, SCI Service
Veterans Administration Medical
  Center
Hampton, VA 23667
(804) 722-9961

Chief, SCI Service
Veterans Administration Medical
  Center
1201 Broad Rock Road
Richmond, VA 23249
(804) 230-0001

Chief, SCI Service
Veterans Administration Medical
  Center

Seattle, WA 98108
(206) 762-1010

Chief, SCI Service
Veterans Administration Medical
  Center
5000 West National Avenue
Wood, WI 53103
(414) 384-2000

VETERANS ADMINISTRATION RESEARCH AND DEVELOPMENT CENTERS AND UNITS

Rehabilitation R&D Center
Veterans Administration Medical
  Center
Hines, IL 60141
(312) 261-6700

Rehabilitation R&D Center
Veterans Administration Medical
  Center

Palo Alto, CA 94304
(415) 493-5000

Rehabilitation Unit
Veterans Administration Medical
  Center
Decatur, GA 30033
(404) 321-6111

OTHER REHABILITATION FACILITIES

Career Counseling and Development
  Services
1739 E. Rose Lane
Phoenix, AZ 85016
(602) 265-6467

Good Samaritan Medical Center
1111 East McDowell Road
P.O. Box 2989
Phoenix, AZ 85062
(602) 239-2000

Casa Colina Hospital for
  Rehabilitation Medicine
255 East Bonita Avenue
Pomona, CA 91767
(714) 593-7521 or (714) 596-7733

Leon S. Peters Rehabilitation Center
Fresno Community Hospital and
  Medical Center
P.O. Box 1232
Fresno, CA 93715
(209) 442-3957

Northridge Hospital Medical Center
18300 Roscoe Boulevard
Northridge, CA 91328
(818) 885-8500

Santa Clara Valley Medical Center
751 South Bascon
San Jose, CA 95128
(408) 299-5643

Sharp Rehabilitation Center
7901 Frost Street
San Diego, CA 92123
(619) 541-3055

Gaylord Hospital
Box 400
Wallingford, CT 06492
(203) 269-3344

National Rehabilitation Hospital
102 Irving Street, N.W.
Washington, DC 20010
(202) 877-1000

Humana Hospital-Lucerne
Lucerne Spinal Injury Center
818 S. Main Lane
Orlando, FL 32801
(305) 237-6148

Memorial Regional Rehabilitation
Center
3599 University Blvd. So.
Jacksonville, FL 32216
(904) 399-6895

Rehabilitation Institute of West
Florida
8391 North Davis Highway
P.O. Box 18900
Pensacola, FL 32523-8900
(904) 474-5358
In Florida 1-800-342-1123

The Tampa General Rehabilitation
Center
Tampa General Hospital
Tampa, FL 33606
(813) 251-7700

University of Miami
School of Medicine
P.O. Box 016960
Miami, FL 32952
(305) 547-6545

Center for Rehabilitation Medicine
Emory University Hospital
1441 Clifton Road N.E.
Atlanta, GA 30322
(404) 727-5512

The Rehabilitation Hospital of the
Pacific
226 N. Kuakini Street
Honolulu, HI 96817
(808) 531-3511

Covenant Medical Center
Rehabilitation Program
2101 Kimball Avenue
Waterloo, IA 50702
(319) 291-3336

Rehabilitation Institute of Chicago
345 E. Superior Street
Chicago, IL 60611
(312) 908-4117

Cardinal Hill Hospital
2020 Versailles Road
Lexington, KY 40504
(606) 254-5701

Louisiana Rehabilitation Institute
Charity Hospital/LM Bldg.
1532 Tulane Avenue
New Orleans, LA 70140
(504) 568-3270

Rehabilitation Institute of New
Orleans
F. Edward Hebert Hospital
1 Sanctuary Drive
New Orleans, LA 70114
(504) 363-2200

Tufts New England Medical Center
171 Harrison Avenue
Boston, MA 02111
(617) 956-7000

Montebello Rehabilitation Hospital
2201 Argonne Drive
Baltimore, MD 21218
(301) 554-5200

The Kennedy Institute for
  Handicapped Children
707 North Broadway
Baltimore, MD 21205
(301) 522-2100

Mayo Clinic
200 1st Street, S.W.
Rochester, MN 55905
(507) 284-2511

Sister Kenny Institute
800 East 28th Street
Minneapolis, MN 55407
(612) 874-4400

University of Minnesota Hospital
860 Mayo Memorial
Box 297
Minneapolis, MN 55440
(612) 626-4050

Spinal Cord Injury Program
Dept. of Rehabilitation Medicine
Jewish Hospital of St. Louis
216 South Kingshighway
St. Louis, MO 63110
(314) 454-7756

UMC–Rusk Rehabilitation Center
501 Rusk Rehabilitation Center
Columbia, MO 65211
(314) 882-3101

Kessler Institute for Rehabilitation
1199 Pleasant Valley Way
West Orange, NJ 07052
(201) 731-3600

Albert Einstein College of Medicine
  of Yeshiva University
1300 Morris Park Avenue
New York, NY 10461
(212) 430-2000

Burke Rehabilitation Center
785 Mamoroneck Avenue
White Plains, NY 10605
(914) 948-0050

Columbia University
College of Physicians and Surgeons
Box 38
630 West 168th Street
New York, NY 10032
(212) 305-3592

Columbia-Presbyterian Medical
  Center
Department of Rehabilitation
  Medicine
622 West 168th Street
New York, NY 10032
(212) 305-2247

Helen Hayes Hospital
SCI Service
Route 9W
West Haverstraw, NY 10993
(914) 947-3000

Cleveland Metropolitan General
Highland View Hospital
3395 Scranton Road
Cleveland, OH 44109
(216) 398-6000

Highland View Hospital
SCI Service
3395 Scranton Road
Cleveland, OH 44109
(216) 459-3483

Ohio State University Hospitals
Dodd Hall
471 Dodd Drive
Columbus, OH 43210
(614) 421-3800

Emanuel Rehabilitation Center
3001 N. Gantenbein Avenue
Portland, OR 97227
(503) 280-4400

Central Pennsylvania SCI Center
Elizabethtown Hospital and
  Rehabilitation Center of the PA
  State University
Elizabethtown, PA 17022
(717) 367-1161

Harmarville Rehabilitation Center
P.O. Box 11460
Guys Run Road
Pittsburgh, PA 15238
(412) 781-5700

Moss Rehabilitation Hospital
12th and Tabor Road
Philadelphia, PA 19141
(215) 329-5715

Piersol Rehabilitation Center
Hospital of University of
  Pennsylvania
3400 Spruce Street
Philadelphia, PA 19104
(215) 662-3242

Baptist Regional Rehabilitation
  Center
1025 Crump Blvd.
Memphis, TN 38104
(901) 522-6585

University of Tennessee
800 Madison Avenue
Memphis, TN 78229
(901) 528-5888

University of Tennessee
  Rehabilitation Engineering Prog.
682 Court Street
Memphis, TN 38163
(901) 528-6445

University of Texas
Health Science Center at Dallas
5323 Harry Hines Blvd.
Dallas, TX 75253-9060
(214) 688-3111

University of Texas
Health Science Center
7703 Floyd Curl Drive
San Antonio, TX 78229
(512) 691-7201

University of Utah Hospital
50 North Medical Drive
Salt Lake City, UT 84132
(801) 581-2121

Medical College of Virginia
Department of Rehabilitation
  Medicine
Box 677
MCV Station
Richmond, VA 23298-0001
(804) 786-0200

Woodrow Wilson Rehabilitation
  Center
Fishersville, VA 22939
(703) 885-9600

Sacred Heart Rehabilitation Hospital
1545 South Layton Blvd.
Milwaukee, WI 53215
(414) 383-4490

Appendix 2. Organizations

PROFESSIONAL AND LAY ORGANIZATIONS

American Academy of Orthotists and Prosthetists, 717 Pendleton Street, Alexandria, VA 22314. Tele. (703) 836-7118. Professional society of certified practitioners in prosthetics and orthotics dedicated to the advancement of the profession and the improvement of patient care. Quarterly publications, *Clinical Prosthetics and Orthotics, Academician;* annual publications, *Membership Directory, Annual Report.*

American Association of Spinal Cord Injury Nurses, 432 Park Avenue South, New York, NY 10016. Tele. (212) 686-6770. Nursing association devoted to the specialized needs of SCI nurses and SCI patients. Quarterly publication, *SCI Nursing.*

American Board for Certification in Orthotics and Prosthetics, Inc., 717 Pendleton Street, Alexandria, VA 22308. Tele. (703) 836-7114. Credentialing and accrediting body for practitioners and facilities qualified to provide health services in orthotics and prosthetics. Quarterly publication, *Mark of Merit.*

American Occupational Therapy Association, 1383 Piccard Drive, Rockville, MD 20850. Tele. (301) 948-9626. Organization of occupational therapy practitioners which accredits occupational therapy education programs, administers national certification examination, represents professionals and consumers before legislative bodies. Monthly publications, *Occupational Therapy News, The American Journal of Occupational Therapy.*

American Orthotic and Prosthetic Association, 717 Pendleton Street, Alexandria, VA 22314. Tele. (703) 836-7116. Trade association composed of members who own and operate patient care facilities for the custom fabrication and fitting of orthoses and prostheses. Monthly magazine, *Almanac;* quarterly scientific journal, *O&P Journal.*

American Paralysis Association (National Office), P.O. Box 187, Short Hills, NJ 07078. Tele. (1-800-225-0292, in NJ 201-379-2690). Encourage and support research to find a cure for paralysis caused by spinal cord injury, head injury, and stroke. Publicize the enormity of spinal cord injury paralysis and the hope for a cure. Quarterly newsletter, *Progress in Research;* journal, *Central Nervous System Trauma* by Mary Ann Liebert, Inc.

American Paraplegia Society, 432 Park Avenue South, New York, NY 10016. Tele. (212) 686-6770. Established to advance, foster, encourage, promote, and improve SCI patient care; to develop and promote research and education related to SCI; and to recognize physicians devoted to the problems of SCI. Quarterly publication, *Journal of the American Paraplegia Society.*

American Physical Therapy Association, 1111 North Fairfax Street, Alexandria, VA 22314. Tele. (703) 684-APTA. Professional organization of physical therapists, assistants, and students to develop and improve physical therapy services and education.

American Spinal Injury Association, Room 619, 250 East Superior Street, Chicago, IL 60611. Tele. (312) 908-3425. Organization of physicians whose primary interest is the care and management of SCI patients. Holds annual scientific meeting open to all. Biannual publication, *ASIA Bulletin;* a number of other publications also are available.

Association for the Advancement of Rehabilitation Technology (RESNA), 1101 Connecticut Avenue, N.W., Suite 700, Washington, DC 20036. Tele. (202) 857-1199. Disabled persons, engineers, therapists, and others interested in promoting the development of devices and products for disabled persons. Quarterly publications, *Rehabilitation Technology Review, RESNA Newsletter;* every 2 years, *Technology for Independent Living Sourcebook;* annual, *Proceedings of the RESNA Annual Conference.*

Canadian Paraplegic Association, 520 Sutherland Dr., Toronto, Canada, M4G 3V9. Tele. (416) 422-5640. Provides services to spinal cord–injured persons through counselling, independent living, and community development programs. Conducts fund raising in support of SCI research. Quarterly journal, *CALIPER.*

Congress of Organizations of the Physically Handicapped, 16630 Beverly Avenue, Tinley Park, IL 60477. Tele. (312) 532-3566. Coalition of organizations of the physically disabled to enhance the quality of lives of persons with a physical disability. Quarterly publication, *COPH Bulletin.*

Dole Foundation for Employment of Persons with Disabilities, 220 Eye Street, N.E., Washington, DC 20002. Tele. (202) 543-6303. Administers funds to establish and operate programs related to employment of disabled persons and sponsors programs, seminars, fellowships, and research activities relating to issues of public policy. Booklet, *Disabled Americans at Work;* brochures, *The Dole Foundation; Guidelines; Grant Announcement Newsletter.*

Help for Incontinent People, P.O. Box 544, Union, SC 29379. Tele. (803) 585-8789. Issues brochures, exercise tapes, and a resource guide of manufacturers' products. Quarterly, *HIP Newsletter.*

Help Them Walk Again Foundation, Inc., 5300 West Charleston Blvd., Las Vegas, NV 89102. Tele. (702) 878-8360. Clinic for spinal cord injuries. Computerized leg trainer, bicycle, and arm stimulator, and full service gym facility. Starting a quarterly newsletter; other publications available.

National Coordinating Council on Spinal Cord Injury, c/o Paralyzed Veterans of America, 801 18th Street, N.W., Washington, DC 20006. Tele. (202) 872-1300. Consortium of lay and professional organizations concerned with spinal cord injury.

National Easter Seal Society, 2023 West Ogden Avenue, Chicago, IL 60612. Tele. (312) 243-8400. Goal is to help people with disabilities attain the greatest degree of independence through self-sufficiency. Bimonthly journal, *Rehabilitation Literature.*

National Organization on Disability, 2100 Pennsylvania Avenue, N.W., Washington, DC 20037. Tele. (202) 293-5960, TTY (202) 293-5968. Promotes and develops the participation of disabled citizens in the life of their communities. Quarterly newsletter, *Report/Update.*

National Rehabilitation Information Center, Catholic University of America, 4407 8th Street, N.E., Washington, DC 20017. Tele. (202) 635-5826 (Voice/TDD); 1-800-34-NARIC (toll free). Rehabilitation information service and research library. Produces two data bases: ABLEDATA (computerized listings of commercially available products) and REHAB-DATA (computerized bibliographic data base of rehabilitation literature and materials). Publishes *Rehabilitation Research Reviews; The Author's Handbook: A Guide to Professional Journals in Rehabilitation; The Periodical List: A Guide to Disability-Related Journals and Newsletters; The Resource Directory: A State Guide to Disability-Related Information.*

National Spinal Cord Injury Association, 149 California Street, Newton, MA 02158. Tele. (617) 964-0521. Addresses SCI issues in the areas of cure and care research, delivery of quality medical care, and living with

SCI. Provides direct services, information and referral, publications, and conferences. Quarterly newsletter, *Spinal Cord Injury Life;* offers a number of other publications as well.

Paralyzed Veterans of America, 801 18th Street, N.W., Washington, DC 20006. Tele. (202) 872-1300.   Thirty-two local chapters and 53 service offices to assist veterans in obtaining benefits. National programs in governmental affairs, medical and research affairs, public education and information, and service. Largest private funding source of spinal cord research in United States through PVA Spinal Cord Research Foundation. Supports conferences, symposia, education programs through PVA Education and Training Foundation. Magazines, *Paraplegia News, Sports N Spokes.*

President's Committee on Employment of the Handicapped, 1111 20th Street, N.W., Room 636, Washington, DC 20036. Tele. (202) 653-5044. Promotes employment opportunities for disabled veterans and handicapped people. Works with public and private sector organizations to develop information and understanding of employment needs and potentials of disabled people. Conducts annual meeting in spring. Annual subscription, *Disabled USA;* other publications also available.

Shake A Leg, P.O. Box 1002, Newport, RI 02840. Tele. (401) 849-8898. Does fund raising and provides programs for SCI persons and related injuries. Programs include sports and recreation, 6-week residential rehabilitation program, and Functional Electrical Stimulation program. Quarterly publication, *Stepping Out.*

Spinal Cord Society, 2410 Lakeview Drive, Fergus Falls, MN 56537. Tele. (218) 739-5252.   Supports and encourages research and treatment targeted upon the cure of spinal cord injury and its associated complications. Monthly newsletter, *Spinal Cord Society Newsletter.*

INDEPENDENT LIVING CENTERS

Alabama

Independent Living Center
3421 Fifth Avenue South
Birmingham, AL 35222
(205) 251-2223

Alaska

Access Alaska
Suite 900
3710 Woodland Drive
Anchorage, AK 99517
(907) 248-4777

Arizona

Arizona Bridge to Independent
  Living (ABIL)
1229 East Washington Street
Phoenix, AZ 85034
(602) 256-ABIL

Arkansas

Independent Living Services Center
5800 Asher Avenue
Little Rock, AR 72204
(501) 568-7588

California

Center for the Independence of the
  Disabled
875 O'Neil Avenue
Belmont, CA 94002
(415) 595-0783

Center for Independent Living
2539 Telegraph Avenue
Berkeley, CA 94704
(415) 841-3900

Northern California Independent
  Living Program
Suite B
555 Rio Lindo Avenue
Chico, CA 95926
(916) 893-8527

California Association for
  Physically Handicapped
Suite 109
1617 E. Saginaw
Fresno, CA 93704
(209) 222-2274
TDD (209) 222-2396

Dayle McIntosh Center for the
  Disabled
Suite 1
8100 Garden Grove Blvd.
Garden Grove, CA 92644
(714) 898-9571

Independent Living Resource
  Center
423 W. Victoria
Santa Barbara, CA 93101
(805) 963-0595

Darrell McDaniel Independent
  Living Center, Inc.
14354 Haynes
Van Nuys, CA 91401
(818) 988-9525

The Center for Independent Living
  of San Gabriel Valley
2231 E. Garvey Avenue
West Covina, CA 91890
(213) 339-1278

Colorado

Center for People with Disabilities
1450 15th Street
Boulder, CO 80302
(303) 442-8662

Atlantis Community, Inc.
Space 18
2200 W. Alameda
Denver, CO 80219
(303) 893-8040

HAIL
Suite 107
1249 East Colfax Ave.
Denver, CO 80218
(303) 831-6381

Helen Campbell Independent
Living Center
835 Colorado Avenue
Grand Junction, CO 81501
(303) 241-0315

Pueblo Goodwill Industries, Inc.
230 N. Union Avenue
Pueblo, CO 81003
(303) 544-9336

Connecticut

Center for Independent Living of
Greater Bridgeport
P.O. Box 3366
Bridgeport, CT 06605
(203) 336-0183

Independence Unlimited
(New Horizons, Inc.)
410 Asylum Street
Hartford, CT 06103
(203) 549-3915

Delaware

Independent Living, Inc.
Liberty Knoll Apartments
Apartment B-1
Route 273
New Castle, DE 19720
(302) 328-1306

District of Columbia

District of Columbia Services for
Independent Living
1400 Florida Avenue, N.E. #3
Washington, DC 20002
(202) 388-0033

Florida

Disability Awareness Now, Inc.
(DAWN)
1001 N.E. 28th Avenue
Gainesville, FL 32601
(904) 377-5141

Center for Survival and
Independent Living (C-SAIL)
Room 101
1310 Northwest 16th Street
Miami, FL 33125
(305) 547-5444

Center for Independent Living
720 N. Denning Drive
Winter Park, FL 32879
(305) 628-2253

Space Coast Association for the
Physically Handicapped
(SCAPH)
Suite 7
P.O. Box 2027
1127 South Patrick Drive
Satellite Beach, FL 32937
(305) 777-2964

Florida Institute for Independent
Living
307 East Seventh Avenue
Tallahassee, FL 32303
(904) 681-6836

Leon Center for Independent
Living
1380 Ocala Road H-4
Tallahassee, FL 32312
(904) 575-9621

Self Reliance
Suite F
12310 N. Nebraska Avenue
Tampa, FL 33612
(813) 977-6368

Georgia

Atlanta Center for Independent
 Living
1201 Glenwood Avenue SE
Atlanta, GA 30316
(404) 656-2952

Hawaii

Vocational Rehabilitation and
 Service for the Blind Division
Department of Social Services
P.O. Box 339
Honolulu, HI 96809
(808) 548-4770

Idaho

Dawn Enterprises, Inc.
P.O. Box 388
Blackfoot, ID 83221
(208) 785-5890

Illinois

Access Living
Suite 525
815 W. Van Buren
Chicago, IL 60607
(312) 226-5900

Kansas

Operation LINK
P.O. Box 1016
Hays, KS 67601
(913) 625-2521

Independence, Inc.
1910 Haskell Avenue
Lawrence, KS 66046
(913) 841-0333

Topeka Resource Center for the
 Handicapped
1119 West 10th
Topeka, KS 66604
(913) 233-6323

Kentucky

Center for Accessible Living
835 W. Jefferson
Louisville, KY 40402
(502) 589-6620

Louisiana

New Horizons Independent Living
 Center
4030 Wallace
Shreveport, LA 71108
(318) 635-3477

Maine

Maine Independent Living Center
74 Winthrop Street
Augusta, ME 04330
(207) 622-5434

Maryland

Maryland Citizens for Housing for
 the Disabled, Inc.
6305-A Sherwood Road
Baltimore, MD 21239
(301) 377-5900

Massachusetts

Stavros Center for Independent
 Living
691 South East Street
Amherst, MA 01002
(413) 256-0473

Boston Center for Independent
 Living
50 New Edgerly Road
Boston, MA 02115
(617) 536-2187

Independence Associates, Inc.
693 Bedford Street
Elmwood, MA 02337
(617) 378-3997

Northeast Independent Living
  Program
Suite 101B
190 Hampshire Street
Lawrence, MA 01840
(617) 687-4288

AD LIB Inc.
442 North Street
Pittsfield, MA 01201
(413) 442-7047

The Center for Living and Working
600 Lincoln Street
Worcester, MA 01605
(617) 853-1068

Michigan

Ann Arbor Center for Independent
  Living
2568 Packard Road
Ann Arbor, MI 48104
(313) 971-0277

Detroit Center for Independent
  Living
Suite 104
4 East Alexandrine Towers
Detroit, MI 48201
(313) 745-9726

Northern Michigan Rural Center
  for Independent Living
Suite 102
209 W. First Street
Gaylord, MI 49735
(517) 732-2448

Grand Rapids Center for
  Independent Living
3375 Division, S.
Grand Rapids, MI 49508
(616) 243-0846

Kalamazoo County Center for
  Independent Living
268 E. Kilgore
Kalamazoo, MI 49001
(616) 345-1516

Center of Handicapper Affairs
Suite C-1
316 N. Capitol Avenue
Lansing, MI 48933
(517) 485-5887 (TTY)

Cristo Rey Hispanic Center for
  Independent Living
1314 Ballard Street
Lansing, MI 48906
(517) 372-4700

Mid-Michigan Urban Center for
  Independent Living
Commission for the Blind
309 N. Washington
P.O. Box 30015
Lansing, MI 48909
(517) 373-9415

Minnesota

Rural Enterprises for Acceptable
  Living, Inc.
244 W. Main Street
Marshall, MN 56258
(507) 532-2221

Rochester Center for Independent
  Living, Inc.
1306 Seventh St., N.W.
Rochester, MN 55901
(507) 285-1815

Metropolitan Center for
  Independent Living, Inc.
1821 University Avenue, N-350
St. Paul, MN 55104
(612) 646-8342

Mississippi

Center for Independent Living
300 Capers Avenue
Jackson, MS 39203
(601) 961-4140

Missouri

Independent Living Center of Mid-
Missouri, Inc.
(Opportunities Unlimited)
111 South Ninth, Suite 211
Columbia, MO 65201
(314) 874-1646

The Whole Person, Inc.
Suite 305E
6301 Rockhill Road
Kansas City, MO 64131
(816) 361-0304

Paraquad, Inc.
4397 Laclede Avenue
St. Louis, MO 63108
(314) 244-3315

Disabled Citizens Alliance for
Independence, Inc.
P.O. Box 675
Viburnum, MO 65566
(314) 244-3315

Montana

Montana Independent Living, Inc.
1301 11th Avenue
Helena, MT 59601
(406) 442-5755

Summit Independent Living Center
1280 South 3rd Street, West
Missoula, MT 59801
(406) 728-1630

Nebraska

League of Human Dignity
Handicap Reach Out, Inc.
Box 948
Chadron, NE 69337
(308) 432-3560

Central NE Goodwill Industries
Goodwill Center for Independent
Living
1804 South Eddy
Grand Island, NE 68801
(308) 384-7896

League of Human Dignity
1423 "O" Street
Lincoln, NE 68508
(402) 474-0820

League of Human Dignity
700½ W. Benjamin
Norfolk, NE 68701
(402) 371-4475

Nevada

Nevada Association for the
Handicapped
6200 West Oakey
Las Vegas, NV 89102
(702) 870-7050

Northern Nevada Center for
Independent Living
790 Sutro Street
Reno, NV 89512
(702) 322-6046

New Jersey

Disabled Information Awareness
and Living (DIAL)
234 Parker Avenue
Clifton, NJ 07011
(201) 340-3700

Handicapped Independence
  Program (HIP)
Social Service Federation
44 Armory Street
Englewood, NJ 07631
(201) 568-0817

New Mexico

New Vistas Independent Living
  Center
St. Michael's Hall
College of Santa Fe
Santa Fe, NM 87501
(505) 473-0550

New York

Capital District Center for
  Independence, Inc. (CDCI)
22 Colvin Avenue
Albany, NY 12206
(518) 459-6422

Western New York Independent
  Living Project
3108 Main Street
Buffalo, NY 14214
(716) 836-0822

Center for Independence of the
  Disabled in New York
Room 611
853 Broadway
New York, NY 10003
(212) 674-2300

Rochester Center for Independent
  Living
464 South Clinton Avenue
Rochester, NY 14620
(716) 546-6990 (TTY)

Westchester Independent Living
  Center
297 Knollwood Road
White Plains, NY 10607
(914) 682-3926 (TTY)

North Carolina

Metrolina Independent Living
  Center
Doctor's Building
Suite G-2
1012 S. Kings Drive
Charlotte, NC 28283
(704) 375-3977

North Dakota

Center for Independent Living
1007 18th Street, N.W.
Mandan, ND 58554
(701) 663-0376

Ohio

Total Living Concepts, Inc.
Suite 101
3333 Vine Street
Cincinnati, OH 45220
(513) 751-1795

Services for Independent Living,
  Inc.
25100 Euclid Avenue
Euclid, OH 44117
(216) 731-1529

Oklahoma

Physically Limited, Inc.
1724 East 8th Street
Tulsa, OK 74104
(918) 592-1235 (TDD)

Oregon

Good Samaritan Hospital
1015 S.W. 22nd Avenue
Portland, OR 97210
(503) 229-7348

Tri-County Independent Living
Program, Inc.
8213 S.E. 17th Avenue
Portland, OR 97212
(503) 230-1225

Pennsylvania

Resources for Living Independently
(RLI)
4721 Pine Street
Philadelphia, PA 19143
(215) 471-2265

Erie Independence House, Inc.
Center for Independent Living
956 W. Second Street
Erie, PA 16507
(814) 459-6161

Three Rivers Center for
Independent Living, Inc.
5129 Penn Avenue
Pittsburgh, PA 15224
(412) 661-3196

Puerto Rico

Centro de Vida Independiente
Box 1681
Hato Rey, PR 00919
(809) 751-5340

Rhode Island

Paraplegia Association of Rhode
Island
Independence Square
500 Prospect Street
Pawtucket, RI 02860
(401) 725-1966

South Carolina

Life Exploration and Alternative
Program (LEAP)
1400 Boston Avenue
West Columbia, SC 29169
(803) 758-8731

South Dakota

Prairie Freedom Center for
Disabled Independence
800 West Avenue, N.
Sioux Falls, SD 57104
(605) 339-6558

Tennessee

Memphis Center for Independent
Living
163 North Angelus
Memphis, TN 38104
(901) 726-6404

Texas

Austin Resource Center for
Independent Living
2818 San Gabriel
Austin, TX 78705
(512) 473-2684

Dallas Center for Independent
Living
8625 King George
Suite 210
Dallas, TX 75235
(214) 631-6900

El Paso Opportunity Center for the
Handicapped
Suite 101
8929 Viscount
El Paso, TX 79925
(915) 591-0800

Houston Center for Independent
Living
The APC Building
6910 Fannin #120
Houston, TX 77030
(713) 795-4252

Independent Living Research
Utilization (ILRU) Project
P.O. Box 20095
Houston, TX 77225

San Antonio Independent Living
Services
416 S. Main Street
San Antonio, TX 78204
(512) 226-0054

Utah

Utah Independent Living Center,
Inc.
764 South 200 West
Salt Lake City, UT 84101
(801) 359-2457 (TTY)

Vermont

Vermont Center for Independent
Living
174 River Street
Montpelier, VT 05602
(802) 229-0501

Virgin Islands

Virgin Islands Association for
Independent Living, Inc.
P.O. Box 3305
Charlotte Amalie
St. Thomas, VI 00801
(809) 774-2740

Virginia

Endependence Center of North
Virginia (ECNV)
4214 9th Street, N.
Arlington, VA 22203
(703) 525-3268

Woodrow Wilson Center for
Independent Living (WWCIL)
P.O. Box 37
Fishersville, VA 22939
(703) 885-9731

Endependence Center, Inc. (ECI)
Plume Center West
100 West Plume Street
Norfolk, VA 23510
(804) 625-3555

Richmond Center for Independent
Living
2900 West Broad Street
Richmond, VA 23230
(804) 353-6503

Washington

Kittitas Community Action
Council, Inc.
115 W. 3rd Street
Ellensburg, WA 98926
(509) 925-1448

Community Home Health Center
190 Queen Anne Avenue North
Seattle, WA 98109
(206) 282-5048

Independent Lifestyle Services-
KCAC
115 W. Third
Ellensburg, WA 98926
(509) 925-1448

West Virginia

Appalachian Council for
Independent Living, Inc.
1427 Lee Street
Charleston, WV 25301
(304) 342-6328

Huntington Center for Independent
Living, Inc.
914½ Fifth Avenue
Huntington, WV 25701
(304) 525-3324

Coordinating Council for
Independent Living, Inc.
1000 Elmer W. Prince Drive
Morgantown, WV 26505
(304) 559-3636

Wisconsin

Access to Independence, Inc.
1954 East Washington Avenue
Madison, WI 53504
(608) 251-7575

Stout Program for Independent
Living—Vocational Development
Center
University of Wisconsin—Stout
Menomonie, WI 54751
(715) 232-2293 (Voice/TTY)

Southeastern Wisconsin Center for
Independent Living, Inc.
(SEWCIL)
Room 522
1545 S. Layton Blvd.
Milwaukee, WI 53215
(414) 643-0910

Wyoming

Independent Living Rehabilitation
550 Rancho Road
Casper, WY 82601
(307) 577-1101

SPORT ORGANIZATIONS

California

Adaptive Programs
Santa Barbara Recreation
Department
P.O. Drawer P-P
Santa Barbara, CA 93102

All Seasons Riding Academy
43510 Osgood Road
Fremont, CA 94539

Bay Area Outreach Recreation
Program
Access Project
605 Eshleman Hall
University of California
Berkeley, CA 94720

California Wheelchair Aviators
Bill Blackwood, Secretary
1117 Rising Hill Way
Escondido, CA 92025

College of Marin
Laurie Lanham MRT
College Avenue
Kentfield, CA 94904

De Anza College
Adaptive Physical Education
21250 Stevens Creek Blvd.
Cupertino, CA 95014

Far West Wheelchair Athletic
Association, Inc.
P.O. Box 26483
San Jose, CA 95159

Handicapped Scuba Association
1104 El Prado
San Clemente, CA 92672

Lake Merritt's Adapted Boating
  Program
Office of Parks and Recreation
1520 Lakeside Drive
Oakland, CA 94612

National Foundation for
  Wheelchair Tennis
1544 Redhill #A
Tustin, CA 92680

Recreation Center for the
  Handicapped
207 Skyline Blvd.
San Francisco, CA 94132

Canada

Sports for the Physically Disabled
333 River Road
Ottawa, Ontario, Canada K1L 8B9

Toronto Bulldogs Wheelchair
  Sports Club
c/o Variety Village
3701 Danforth Avenue
Scarborough, Ontario
M1N 2G2 Canada

Colorado

Aspen Handicap Skiers Association
Ed Lucks Institute
P.O. Box 5429
0174 Meadow Road
Snowmass Village, CO 81615

Breckenridge Outdoor Education
  Center
P.O. Box 697
Breckenridge, CO 80424

Children's Hospital
Handicapped Sports Program
1056 East 19th Avenue
Denver, CO 80218

Durango Purgatory Handicapped
  Sports Association
175 Beatrice Drive
Durango, CO 81301

Horizons
P.O. Box 772143
Steamboat Springs, CO 80477

National Handicapped Sports and
  Recreation Association
Competition Office
Capitol Hill Station
P.O. Box 18664
Denver, CO 80218

National Wheelchair Athletic
  Association
Suite C
2107 Templeton Gap Road
Colorado Springs, CO 80907

Rocky Mountain Handicapped
  Sportsman's Association
P.O. Box 18036
Denver, CO 80218

District of Columbia

National Handicapped Sports and
  Recreation Association
Farragut Station
P.O. Box 33141
Washington, DC 20033

Iowa

Special Recreation, Inc.
362 Koser Avenue
Iowa City, IA 52240

Idaho

Recreation Unlimited, Inc.
P.O. Box 447
Boise, ID 83702

Illinois

Chicagoland Handicapped Skiers
RRI, Box 115B
Sandwich, IL 60548

Kentucky

National Wheelchair Basketball
 Assoc.
University of Kentucky
110 Seaton Building
Lexington, KY 40506

Union Aviation, Inc.
P.O. Box 207
Sturgis, KY 42459

Massachusetts

New England Sportsmen's
 Association
P.O. Box 2150
Boston, MA 02106

Wheelchair Motorcycle Association
101 Torey Street
Brockton, MA 02401

Minnesota

Courage Alpine Skiers
c/o Courage Center
3915 Golden Valley Road
Golden Valley, MN 55427

Courage Center
3016 Golden Valley Road
Golden Valley, MN 00422

Vinland National Center
P.O. Box 308
Loretto, MN 55357

Voyageur Outward Bound School
P.O. Box 250
Long Lake, MN 55356

Wilderness Inquiry II
Suite 327a
1313 Fifth St., S.E.
Minneapolis, MN 55414

Nevada

City of Las Vegas
Department of Recreation and
 Leisure Activities
749 Veterans Memorial Drive
Las Vegas, NV 89101

New Mexico

Soaring Society of America, Inc.
P.O. Box E
Hobbs, NM 88240

New York

The Silver Wheelchair Football
127 Farmingdale
Ckeektowaga, NY 14225

USA Wheelchair Sports Fund
Suite 29
1550 Franklin Avenue
Mineola, NY 11501

Ohio

Indoor Sports, Inc.
1145 Highland Street
Napoleon, OH 43545

Kinesiotherapy Clinic
University of Toledo
2801 West Bancroft Street
Toledo, OH 43606

Three Trackers of Ohio
3655 Brush Road
Richfield, OH 44286

Oregon

All Outdoors, Inc.
P.O. Box 1100
Redmond, OR 97756

Flying Outriggers Ski Club
Shared Outdoor Adventure
  Recreation (SOAR)
211 Oregon Pioneer Bldg.
P.O. Box 14583
Portland, OR 97204-2672

Mobility International USA
P.O. Box 3551
Eugene, OR 97403

Pennsylvania

National Foundation for Happy
  Horsemanship for the
  Handicapped, Inc.
P.O. Box 462
Malvern, PA 19355

Texas

Freedom Flyers, Inc.
P.O. Box 479
Rowlett, TX 75088

Peter Burwash International Special
  Programs
Suite 126
2203 Timberloch Place
The Woodlands, TX 77380

Vermont

Vermont Association for
  Handicapped
A. M. Dirmaier
1232 Route 2
Willston, VT

Wisconsin

Rollin Warhawk Wheelchair
  Basketball Camp and Coaching
  Clinic
Roseman Bldg.
1004 University of Wisconsin
Whitewater, WI 53190

Whitewater Rollin Warhawk
  Athletics
University of Wisconsin—
  Whitewater
1004 Roseman Bldg.
Whitewater, WI 53190

PARALYZED VETERANS OF AMERICA SERVICE OFFICES

National service office:

Paralyzed Veterans of America
801 18th Street, N.W.
Washington, DC 20006
(202) 872-1300

National appeals office:

Paralyzed Veterans of America
Shoreham Building
VACO (817A)
806 15th Street, N.W.
Washington, DC 20420
(202) 347-1911

Paralyzed Veterans of America
Montgomery Veterans Administration
  Regional Office
Room 335
474 S. Court Street
Montgomery, AL 36104
(205) 832-7222

Paralyzed Veterans of America
Little Rock Veterans Administration
  Regional Office
Room 107
1200 West 3rd Street
Little Rock, AR 72201
(501) 378-6068

Paralyzed Veterans of America
Phoenix Veterans Administration
  Regional Office
Suite 619
3225 North Central Avenue
Phoenix, AZ 85012
(602) 241-2700, 274-4924

Paralyzed Veterans of America
Los Angeles Veterans Administration
  Regional Office
Federal Building, Room 5208
11000 Wilshire Boulevard
Los Angeles, CA 90024
(213) 209-7796

Paralyzed Veterans of America
San Diego Veterans Administration
  Regional Office
2022 Camino Del Rio North
San Diego, CA 92108
(619) 293-5557, 260-1025

Paralyzed Veterans of America
San Francisco Veterans
  Administration Regional Office
Room 1204-A
211 Main Street
San Francisco, CA 94105
(415) 957-1617

Paralyzed Veterans of America
Veterans Administration Regional
  Office
44 Union Blvd.
Box 25126
Denver, CO 80225
(303) 980-2899

Paralyzed Veterans of America
Hartford Veterans Administration
  Regional Office
450 Main Street
Hartford, CT 06103
(203) 722-2506/08

Paralyzed Veterans of America
Washington Veterans Administration
  Regional Office
Room 1201-C
941 North Capitol Street, N.E.
Washington, DC 20421
(202) 275-0241

Paralyzed Veterans of America
Wilmington Veterans Administration
  Regional Office
Room 18
1601 Kirkwood Highway
Wilmington, DE 19805
(302) 994-2511, Ext. 325

Paralyzed Veterans of America
Veterans Administration Medical
  Center
Bay Pines Boulevard, N.
Bay Pines, FL 33504
(813) 398-6661, Ext. 4905

Paralyzed Veterans of America
Gainesville Veterans Administration
  Medical Center
Room B-241
Gainesville, FL 32602
(904) 376-6111, Ext. 6031

Paralyzed Veterans of America
Veterans Administration Outpatient
Clinic
Room 47
5599 N. Dixie Highway
Oakland Park, FL 33334
(305) 771-2101, Ext. 34

Paralyzed Veterans of America
Veterans Administration Outpatient
Clinic
83 W. Columbia Road
Orlando, FL 32806
(305) 425-7521, Ext. 189

Paralyzed Veterans of America
P.O. Box 31365
St. Petersburg, FL 33732-1365
(813) 893-3293/3442/3443

Paralyzed Veterans of America
James A. Haley Veterans
Administration Medical Center
Room A-246
13000 North 30th Street
Tampa, FL 33612
(813) 972-2000, Ext. 6594/6595

Paralyzed Veterans of America
Veterans Administration Regional
Office, Room 207
730 Peachtree St., N.E.
Atlanta, GA 30365
(404) 347-4611/7845

Paralyzed Veterans of America
Augusta Veterans Administration
Medical Center
Downtown Division, Room 2C-100
950 15th Street
Augusta, GA 30910
(404) 823-2219

Paralyzed Veterans of America
Chicago Veterans Administration
Regional Office, Suite 488
536 South Clark Street
Chicago, IL 60605
(312) 663-1872

Paralyzed Veterans of America
Indianapolis Veterans Administration
Regional Office, Room 170
575 N. Pennsylvania Street
Indianapolis, IN 46204
(317) 634-1407 or 269-2764

Paralyzed Veterans of America
Wichita Veterans Administration
Regional Office, Room 170
901 George Washington Blvd.
Wichita, KS 67211
(316) 269-6290 or 262-6937

Paralyzed Veterans of America
Louisville Veterans Administration
Regional Office, Room 554-D
600 Federal Place
Louisville, KY 40202
(502) 582-5085

Paralyzed Veterans of America
New Orleans Veterans Administration
Regional Office
Room 9021
701 Loyola Avenue
New Orleans, LA 70113
(504) 589-6068/6401

Paralyzed Veterans of America
Boston Veterans Administration
Regional Office
JFK Federal Building, Room 326
Boston, MA 02203
(617) 223-3304

Paralyzed Veterans of America
Veterans Administration Regional
Office
Federal Building, Room GO-7D
31 Hopkins Plaza
Baltimore, MD 21201
(301) 962-3908

Paralyzed Veterans of America
McNamara Federal Building, Room
1233
477 Michigan Avenue
Detroit, MI 48226
(313) 961-9583

Paralyzed Veterans of America
Veterans Administration Regional
  Office
Federal Building, Room 194B
Ft. Snelling, MN 55111
(612) 726-6442

Paralyzed Veterans of America
Jackson Veterans Administration
  Regional Office
Room 117
100 West Capitol
Jackson, MS 39269
(601) 965-5795

Paralyzed Veterans of America
St. Louis Veterans Administration
  Regional Office
Room 4015
1520 Market Street
St. Louis, MO 63103
(314) 425-5921

Paralyzed Veterans of America
Lincoln Veterans Administration
  Regional Office
Room 128
100 Centennial Mall North
Lincoln, NB 68508
(402) 471-5017

Paralyzed Veterans of America
Winston-Salem Veterans
  Administration Regional Office
Room 429
251 N. Main Street
Winston-Salem, NC 27155
(919) 761-3189

Paralyzed Veterans of America
Newark Veterans Administration
  Regional Office
20 Washington Place
Newark, NJ 07102
(201) 645-6068

Paralyzed Veterans of America
P.O. Box 1105
Albuquerque, NM 87103
(505) 766-3447

Paralyzed Veterans of America
Buffalo Veterans Administration
  Regional Office
Federal Building
111 West Huron Street
Buffalo, NY 14202
(716) 856-6582

Paralyzed Veterans of America
Castle Point Veterans Administration
  Medical Center
Castle Point, NY 12511
(914) 831-2000, ext. 5195

Paralyzed Veterans of America
New York Veterans Administration
  Regional Office
252 Seventh Avenue
New York, NY 10001
(212) 924-7230

Paralyzed Veterans of America
Cleveland Veterans Administration
  Regional Office
Room 1017
1240 East Ninth Street
Cleveland, OH 44199
(216) 522-3214 or 522-7709

Paralyzed Veterans of America
Muskogee Veterans Administration
  Regional Office
Room 3D04
125 South Main Street
Muskogee, OK 74401
(918) 687-2183/2184

Paralyzed Veterans of America
Portland Veterans Administration
  Regional Office
Federal Building, Room 1440
1220 Southwest Third
Portland, OR 97204
(503) 221-4096/3167

Paralyzed Veterans of America
Philadelphia Veterans Administration
  Regional Office
5000 Wissahickon Avenue
Philadelphia, PA 19101
(215) 951-5410

Paralyzed Veterans of America
Pittsburgh Veterans Administration
  Regional Office
Federal Building, Room 431
1000 Liberty Avenue
Pittsburgh, PA 15222
(412) 644-6794/6467

Paralyzed Veterans of America
San Juan Veterans Administration
  Regional Office
Room 153-A
G.P.O. Box 4867
San Juan, PR 00936
(809) 780-3840 (home)

Paralyzed Veterans of America
Columbia Veterans Administration
  Regional Office
Room 216
1801 Assembly Street
Columbia, SC 29201
(803) 765-5758/5757

Paralyzed Veterans of America
Veterans Administration Medical and
  Regional Office Center
2501 W. 22nd Street
P.O. Box 5046
Sioux Falls, SD 57117
(605) 336-2980, Ext. 445

Paralyzed Veterans of America
Memphis Veterans Administration
  Medical Center
Room 405
1030 Jefferson Avenue
Memphis, TN 38104
(901) 523-8990, Ext. 5666/5667

Paralyzed Veterans of America
Nashville Veterans Administration
  Regional Office
Room A361
110 9th Avenue South
Nashville, TN 37203
(615) 736-7713/7714

Paralyzed Veterans of America
Houston Veterans Administration
  Regional Office
2515 Murworth Drive
Houston, TX 77054
(713) 660-4095/4096/4097

Paralyzed Veterans of America
Waco Veterans Administration
  Regional Office
1400 North Valley Mills Drive
Waco, TX 76799
(817) 757-6438

Paralyzed Veterans of America
Service Office
Veterans Administration Medical
  Center
Room 1U148
1201 Broad Rock Blvd.
Richmond, VA 23249
(804) 230-0001, Ext. 2740

Paralyzed Veterans of America
Roanoke Veterans Administration
  Regional Office
Room 1133
210 Franklin Road, S.W.
Roanoke, VA 24011
(703) 343-7388

Paralyzed Veterans of America
Seattle Veterans Administration
  Regional Office, Room 1048
915 Second Avenue
Seattle, WA 98174
(206) 442-2689

Paralyzed Veterans of America
901 S.W. 152nd St.
Seattle, WA 98166
(206) 241-1843/7016

Paralyzed Veterans of America
American Lake Veterans
  Administration Medical Center
Tacoma, WA 98493
(206) 582-8440, Ext. 6990

Paralyzed Veterans of America
Veterans Administration Regional
Office
Zablocki Veterans Administration
Center
(5000 West National Avenue, Bldg. 6)
P.O. Box 6
Milwaukee, WI 53295
(414) 671-8289/8290

Paralyzed Veterans of America
Veterans Administration Regional
Office, Room 216
640 4th Avenue
Huntington, WV 25701
(304) 529-5303

VETERANS ADMINISTRATION REGIONAL OFFICES

Veterans Administration Regional
Office
235 East 8th Avenue
Anchorage, AK 99501

Veterans Administration Regional
Office
474 South Court Street
Montgomery, AL 36104

Veterans Administration Regional
Office
1200 West 3rd Street
Little Rock, AR 72201

Veterans Administration Regional
Office
3225 North Central Avenue
Phoenix, AZ 85102

Veterans Administration Regional
Office
Federal Building
11000 Wilshire Blvd.
Los Angeles, CA 90024

Veterans Administration Regional
Office
2022 Camino Del Rio North
San Diego, CA 92108

Veterans Administration Regional
Office
211 Main Street
San Francisco, CA 94105

Veterans Administration Regional
Office
U.S. Veterans Administration
APO, San Francisco, CA 96528
(for Manila, the Philippines)

Veterans Administration Regional
Office
44 Union Blvd.
P.O. Box 25126
Denver, CO 80225

Veterans Administration Regional
Office
450 Main St.
Hartford, CT 06103

Veterans Administration Regional
Office
941 North Capitol St., N.E.
Washington, DC 20421

Veterans Administration Medical and
Regional Office Center
1601 Kirkwood Highway
Wilmington, DE 19805

Veterans Administration Regional
Office
144 First Avenue, S.
P.O. Box 1437
St. Petersburg, FL 33731

Veterans Administration Regional
Office
730 Peachtree St., N.E.
Atlanta, GA 30365

Veterans Administration Regional
Office
P.O. Box 50188
Honolulu, HI 96850

Veterans Administration Regional
Office
210 Walnut Street
Des Moines, IA 50309

Veterans Administration Regional
Office
Federal Building and U.S.
Courthouse
550 West Fort Street
P.O. Box 044
Boise, ID 83724

Veterans Administration Regional
Office
536 South Clark Street
P.O. Box 8136
Chicago, IL 60680

Veterans Administration Regional
Office
575 North Pennsylvania Street
Indianapolis, IN 46204

Veterans Administration Medical and
Regional Office Center
901 George Washington Blvd.
Wichita, KS 67211

Veterans Administration Regional
Office
600 Federal Place
Louisville, KY 40202

Veterans Administration Regional
Office
701 Loyola Avenue
New Orleans, LA 70113

Veterans Administration Regional
Office
John F. Kennedy Building
Government Center
Boston, MA 02203

Veterans Administration Regional
Office
Federal Building
31 Hopkins Plaza
Baltimore, MD 21201

Veterans Administration Medical and
Regional Office Center
Togus, ME 04330

Veterans Administration Regional
Office
Patrick V. McNamara Federal
Building
477 Michigan Avenue
Detroit, MI 48226

Veterans Administration Regional
Office and Insurance Center
Federal Building
Fort Snelling
St. Paul, MN 55111

Veterans Administration Regional
Office
Federal Building
1520 Market Street
St. Louis, MO 63103

Veterans Administration Regional
Office
100 West Capitol Street
Jackson, MS 39269

Veterans Administration Medical and
Regional Office Center
Fort Harrison, MT 59636

Veterans Administration Regional
Office
Federal Building
251 North Main Street
Winston-Salem, NC 27155

Veterans Administration Medical and
Regional Office Center
655 First Avenue, N.
Fargo, ND 58102

Veterans Administration Regional
Office
Federal Building
100 Centennial Mall, N.
Lincoln, NE 68508

Veterans Administration Regional
Office
Norris Cotton Federal Building
275 Chestnut Street
Manchester, NH 03103

Veterans Administration Regional
Office
20 Washington Place
Newark, NJ 07102

Veterans Administration Regional
Office
Dennis Chavez Federal Building
U.S. Courthouse
500 Gold Avenue, S.W.
Albuquerque, NM 87102

Veterans Administration Regional
Office
245 East Liberty Street
Reno, NV 89520

Veterans Administration Regional
Office
Federal Building
111 West Huron Street
Buffalo, NY 14202

Veterans Administration Regional
Office
252 Seventh Avenue at 24th Street
New York, NY 10001

Veterans Administration Regional
Office
Anthony J. Celebrezze Federal
Building
1240 East Ninth Street
Cleveland, OH 44199

Veterans Administration Regional
Office
Federal Building
125 South Main Street
Muskogee, OK 74401

Veterans Administration Regional
Office
Federal Building
1220 Southwest 3rd Avenue
Portland, OR 97204

Veterans Administration Regional
Office and Insurance Center
P.O. Box 8079
Philadelphia, PA 19101

Veterans Administration Regional
Office
1000 Liberty Avenue
Pittsburgh, PA 15222

Veterans Administration Medical and
Regional Office Center
GPO Box 4867
San Juan, PR 00936

Veterans Administration Regional
Office
380 Westminster Mall
Providence, RI 02903

Veterans Administration Regional
Office
1801 Assembly Street
Columbia, SC 29201

Veterans Administration Medical and
Regional Office Center
Royal C. Johnson Veterans Memorial
Hospital
2501 West 22nd St.
Sioux Falls, SD 57117

Veterans Administration Regional
Office
110 Ninth Avenue, S.
Nashville, TN 37203

Veterans Administration Regional
Office
2515 Murworth Drive
Houston, TX 77054

Veterans Administration Regional
Office
1400 North Valley Mills Drive
Waco, TX 76799

Veterans Administration Regional
Office
Federal Building
125 South State Street
Salt Lake City, UT 84147

Veterans Administration Regional
Office
210 Franklin Road, S.W.
Roanoke, VA 24011

Veterans Administration Medical and
Regional Office Center
White River Junction, VT 05001

Veterans Administration Regional
Office
Federal Building
915 Second Avenue
Seattle, WA 98174

Veterans Administration Regional
Office
P.O. Box 6
Milwaukee, WI 53193

Veterans Administration Regional
Office
640 Fourth Avenue
Huntington, WV 25701

Veterans Administration Medical and
Regional Office Center
2360 East Pershing Blvd.
Cheyenne, WY 82001

Appendix 3. NIDRR

NIDRR RESEARCH AND TRAINING CENTERS

Center	Service
University of Alabama at Birmingham Department of Rehabilitation Medicine University Station Birmingham, AL 35294	Spinal cord dysfunction
University of Arkansas Rehabilitation Research and Training Center 346 North West Avenue Fayetteville, AR 72701 (501) 575-3656	Vocational aspects of rehabilitation
Rancho Los Amigos Hospital Professional Staff Association 7413 Golondrinas Street Downey, CA 90242 (213) 922-7402	Aging
University of California at Davis Office of Research 275 Mrak Hall Davis, CA 95616 (916) 752-2903	Management of neuromuscular disease
George Washington University Rice Hall, 6th Floor Washington, DC 20052 (202) 676-2624	Psychosocial environment and social and attitudinal barriers

Center	Service
The Menninger Foundation Jayhawk Towers, 9th Floor 700 Jackson Topeka, KS 66603 (913) 233-2051	Vocational rehabilitation
University of Kansas Bureau of Child Research 223 Haworth Lawrence, KS 66045 (913) 864-4950	Independent living services

Tufts—New England Medical Center,
  Inc.
Department of Rehabilitation
  Medicine
171 Harrison Avenue
Boston, MA 02111
(617) 955-5622
	Musculoskeletal disorders in children
	  and adults

Albert Einstein College of Medicine/
  Yeshiva University
Multiple Sclerosis Comprehensive
  Care Center
1300 Morris Park
New York, NY 10461
(212) 430-2682
	Multiple sclerosis

Human Resources Center I.U. Willets Road Albertson, NY 11507 (516) 747-5400	Research on employability of disabled persons
New York University Medical Center School of Medicine 550 First Avenue New York, NY 10016 (212) 340-6105	Research on management of neuromuscular disease
Syracuse University Center on Human Policy 4E Huntington Hall Syracuse, NY 13210 (315) 423-3851	Community integration and resource support

Center	Service
University of Pennsylvania Department of Physical Medicine and Rehabilitation 3451 Walnut Street Philadelphia, PA 19104 (215) 662-3261	Aging
Baylor College of Medicine Department of Rehabilitation 1200 Moursund Avenue Houston, TX 77030 (713) 797-1440, ext. 477	Rehabilitation of SCI persons
The Institute for Rehabilitation and Research Independent Living Research Utilization P.O. Box 20095 Houston, TX 77030 (713) 799-7011	Independent living needs
West Virginia University West Virginia Rehabilitation Research and Training Center Suite E One Dunbar Plaza Dunbar, WV 25064-3098 (304) 766-7138	Management of vocational rehabilitation services

NIDRR PROJECTS

Center	Service
Columbia University School of Social Work—Box 20 Low Memorial Library New York, NY 10027 (212) 280-5173	Disabled workers and their jobs: Managing continued employment
Rehabilitation International 432 Park Avenue South New York, NY 10016 (212) 679-6520	Rehabilitation international

Center	Service
World Rehabilitation Fund 400 East 34th Street New York, NY 10016 (216) 679-2934	International exchange of experts and information in rehabilitation
Case Western Reserve University School of Medicine 2119 Abington Road Cleveland, OH 44106 (216) 444-4900	Functional electrical stimulation
The Institute for Rehabilitation and Research Independent Living Service Delivery Project P.O. Box 20095 Houston, TX 77225 (713) 797-1440, Ext. 504	Rural independent living
National Association of Partners of the Americas, Inc. PATH Americas Program 1424 K Street, N.W. Washington, DC 20005 (202) 628-3300	Handicapped children and adults
Johns Hopkins University Division of Education 3400 North Charles Street Baltimore, MD 21218 (301) 338-8273	Microcomputer technology for severely disabled
ABT Associates, Inc. 55 Wheeler Street Cambridge, MA 02138 (617) 492-7100	Functional assessment in vocational rehabilitation—validation and application
University of Nebraska at Lincoln Human Development/Families Department Home Economics 140 Lincoln, NE 68583-0809 (402) 472-3910	Self-help videotapes for disabled

Center	Service
Albert Einstein College of Medicine/ Yeshiva University Multiple Sclerosis Comprehensive Care Center 1300 Morris Park Avenue New York, NY 10461 (212) 430-2682	Research on multiple sclerosis
Human Interaction Research Institute Suite 1120 10889 Wilshire Blvd. Los Angeles, CA 90024 (213) 879-1373	Improving utilization of research results
Catholic University of America National Rehabilitation Information Center (NARIC) 4407 Eighth St., N.E. Washington, DC 20017 (202) 635-5822	Information services for the rehabilitation community
Electronic Industries Foundation Suite 700 1901 Pennsylvania Avenue, N.W. Washington, DC 20006 (202) 955-5823	Development of a national rehabilitation engineering service delivery system
Howard University School of Education 2400 6th St., N.W. Washington, DC 20059 (202) 686-6726	Model to improve rehabilitation to urban minority groups
Planning Systems International, Inc. Suite 104 200 Little Falls Street Falls Church, VA 22046 (703) 533-0383	Publishes *Rehab Briefs*—findings of NIDRR research
Virginia Department of Rehabilitation Services 4901 Fitzhugh Avenue P.O. Box 11045 Richmond, VA 23230 (804) 257-0264	Economics of disability

Western Washington University
School of Education
Bellingham, WA 98225
(206) 676-3319

Rural independent living network

NIDRR FIELD INITIATED RESEARCH

Center	Service
Rancho Los Amigos Hospital, Inc. Professional Staff Association 7413 Golondrinas Street Downey, CA 90242 (213) 922-8111	Long-term neurological change in SCI
Craig Hospital 3425 South Clarkson Englewood, CO 80110 (303) 789-8214	Collaborative study of high quadriplegia
George Washington University Office of Sponsored Research Rice Hall, 6th Floor Washington, DC 20052 (202) 676-8650	Social skills training
Illinois Institute of Technology Pritzker Institute of Medical Engineering IIT Center Chicago, IL 60616 (312) 567-5324	Restoring leg function with implantable orthoses
Rehabilitation Institute of Chicago Rehabilitation Research and Training Center 345 East Superior Chicago, IL 60611 (312) 492-3327	Urinary tract infection in SCI persons—dip-slide bladder irrigation techniques
University of Illinois at Chicago Evaluation Division Institute F/T Study DD 1640 West Roosevelt Road Chicago, IL 60608 (312) 996-1647	Longitudinal study of public expenditures for services for disabled

Center	Service

Purdue University
Department of Agricultural
  Engineering
West Lafayette, IN 47907
(317) 494-1191
	Information resource base for
	  disabled farm operators and
	  agricultural workers

Boston University
Sarget College/Allied Health
  Professions
25 Buick Street
Boston, MA 02215
(617) 353-3549
	Promoting the rehabilitation of the
	  psychiatrically disabled/community
	  research services

Michigan State University
Community Health Sciences
East Lansing, MI 48824
(517) 355-1824
	Study disability management and
	  rehabilitation programs of specific
	  employers in Michigan

Columbia University
School of Social Work
Industrial Social Welfare Center
Box 20
Low Memorial Library
New York, NY 10027
(212) 280-5173
	Promoting rehabilitation services and
	  policies—work site-based EAPs as
	  effective advocates

SUNY Research Foundation of
  Buffalo
P.O. Box 9
Albany, NY 12201
	National data base for medical
	  rehabilitation

International Center for Industry Labor and Rehabilitation P.O. Box 714 Dublin, OH 43017 (614) 889-0781	Study factors creating work disability in the older worker
Thomas Jefferson University 11th and Walnut Streets Philadelphia, PA 19107 (215) 928-6573	Functional recovery of wrist extensors after quadriplegia

Center	Service
Baylor College of Medicine Department of Rehabilitation 1200 Moursund Avenue Houston, TX 77030 (713) 799-7035	Materials for percutaneous passage
University of Washington Rehabilitation Medicine RJ-30 BB919 Health Science Bldg. Seattle, WA 98185	Rehabilitation of arm and hand weakness due to upper motor neuron disease

NIDRR INNOVATION GRANTS

Center	Service
Department of Human Services Division of Rehabilitation Services— Arkansas 1401 Brookwood Dr. P.O. Box 3781 Little Rock, AR 72203 (501) 371-7596	Create an awareness of rehabilitation technology
Southern Illinois University Rehabilitation Institute Carbondale, IL 62901 (618) 536-7704	Independent living skills
Purdue University Division of Sponsored Programs West Lafayette, IN 49707 (317) 494-1191	Modified agricultural equipment
University of Kansas Bureau of Child Research 223 Haworth Lawrence, KS 66045 (913) 864-4295	Form statewide coalition of self-help groups and access resources for families
Rutgers University Department of Economics New Brunswick, NJ 08903 (201) 932-7891	Feasibility study for center on policy research

Center	Service
National Association for Industry Education Cooperation 235 Hendricks Blvd. Buffalo, NY 14226 (716) 834-7047	Participation of handicapped persons in apprenticeship: the state of the art
Washington State University Cooperative Extension Room 411, Agricultural Sciences Bldg. Pullman, WA 99164-6230 (206) 593-8547	Recovery, rehabilitation, and reemployment of injured workers in Washington State

Appendix 4. Glossary

Adaptive equipment. Devices that assist you in doing what you want to do.

ADL. Activities of daily living, such as getting dressed, bathing, cooking, and brushing your teeth.

Ambulate. To walk.

Astrocyte. A type of cell that appears in the central nervous system.

Autonomic dysreflexia (hyperreflexia). Reaction of the autonomic nervous system to noxious stimuli, such as infection, bladder distension, or irritation from an improperly placed catheter. Symptoms include flushing, chills, headache or pounding sensation, high blood pressure, and increased spasticity.

Autonomic nervous system. The part of the nervous system that includes involuntary functions.

Axon. Projection from the cell body which carries messages out of the nerve cell.

Bedsore. *See* Decubitus ulcer.

Biofeedback. Using technology to monitor involuntary body processes (i.e., blood pressure, skin temperature, heart beat) to enable an individual to control them consciously. Information is usually provided through the person's sense of hearing or sight.

Bladder. Part of the urinary tract which holds body waste products (urine).

Bladder irrigation. Method of sending a liquid solution via a catheter into the bladder to flush the bladder out.

Bony prominence. Bone which comes close to the outer skin of the body without having a thick layer of fatty tissue to protect it.

Bowel care. A system of managing and stimulating the bowels to ensure regular bowel movements.

Brace. A device used to support a body part and keep it in the correct position.

Brown Sequard syndrome. Caused by damage to one-half of the spinal cord. It results in loss of sensation on the same side of the lesion and loss of pain and temperature senses on the opposite side.

Calcification. The action by which there is hardening of tissue due to the collection of insoluble calcium salts.

Calculi. Also called stones. They are an accumulation of body salts and may occur as bladder or kidney stones.

Canadian crutch. Type of crutch comprised of two supports reaching halfway between the elbow and shoulder, with a hand bar and curved upper arm which bears the user's weight.

Catheter. An instrument used to empty a body cavity of fluid (i.e., empty the bladder of urine).

Cervical. Relates to the neck or cervix.

CNS. Central nervous system. System of the body which contains the brain and spinal cord.

Coccyx. The end of the spinal column; often called tailbone.

Colostomy. A surgical procedure which provides an artificial anus.

Complete lesion. An injury where no messages get through the injured part of the spinal cord resulting in total loss of muscle power and sensation below the level of injury.

Compression. Type of spinal injury where pressure is exerted on the spinal cord by bone fragments which crush the spinal cord and results in motor and sensory loss.

Contracture. Refers to a shortening of the muscle which may result in stiffness of the joints (i.e., hips, knees, ankles).

Contusion. Bruise or injury to tissue. In the spinal cord, this type of injury may result in temporary or permanent damage below the level of injury.

Crede'. A technique of applying pressure to the lower abdomen to empty the bladder of urine.

Cystometrogram. Measurement of the pressure of forces affecting the bladder and the bladder's capacity to withstand pressure.

Cystoscopy. Examination of the interior of the bladder by means of an instrument called a cystoscope.

Decubitus ulcer. Skin and tissue breakdown due to prolonged pressure on the skin which disrupts the flow of blood to susceptible areas (i.e., those areas of the body which support a person's weight). Also known as bedsores and pressure sores.

Derma. Another name for skin.

Detrusor muscle. Located in the bladder; enables the bladder to contract.

Dialysis. *See* Hemodialysis. Procedure performed using a machine to filter the body's waste products which accumulate in the bloodstream. This procedure may be used when the kidneys can no longer perform this function.

Diaphragm. Muscle between the chest and abdominal cavity which facilitates respiration.

Distension. The act of or state of being abnormally stretched beyond capacity.

Diuretic. To increase the flow of urine by using drugs.

Dysreflexia. *See* Autonomic dysreflexia.

Dyssynergia. Disruption of the coordination that occurs between the urinary sphincters and the bladder to empty the bladder of urine.

Environmental control unit. Type of system which enables a severely physically disabled person to operate different electrical devices in their environment (i.e., lamps, telephone, television, bed).

Fecal impaction. Blockage of the bowels resulting in severe constipation.

FES (functional electrical stimulation). Term used to describe several methods for improving function in paralyzed limbs by stimulating nerves and muscles.

Flat plate. X-ray taken of the abdomen.

FNS (functional neuromuscular stimulation). *See* FES.

Gizmo. A piece of equipment used externally by males to collect urine; also called a Texas catheter.

Glial cells. Cells that surround the nerve cells and appear to control the life and growth of nerve cells.

Gray matter. One of the major sections of the spinal cord which is shaped like an H and is comprised of millions of nerve cells.

Hemodialysis. *See* Dialysis. The process of purifying the blood by dialysis.

Heterotopic ossification. An excess of bone produced near the joint which may result in restricted movement.

Homeostasis. A balance or state of equilibrium between different components of an organism.

Hydronephrosis. Stretching of the kidney resulting from reflux or pressure in the bladder.

Hypotonic bladder. Muscles in the bladder stay relaxed due to spinal cord damage and contractions are not strong enough to empty the bladder.

Ileal loop/ileal diversion. Procedure performed surgically in which the ureters are placed in an artificial channel (called a conduit) which runs through the abdominal wall and a permanent opening made for urine to pass outside the body.

Incomplete lesion. An injury where some messages are able to get through the spinal cord after injury and so some motor control and sensation may remain.

Indwelling catheter. A catheter which is left in the bladder to empty the bladder of urine.

Intercostal muscles.　Located between the ribs, these muscles regulate the diameter of the chest cage.

Intervertebral discs.　Tough gristle "cushions" that separate the spinal vertebrae.

Ischemia.　Deficiency of blood cells to tissue due to the blockage of blood flow.

Ischium.　Two bones which protrude in the buttocks.

IVP (intravenous pyelogram).　X-ray taken after injecting a dye into the vein which outlines the urinary system.

KAFO (knee ankle foot orthosis).　Bracing system used to enable some spinal cord–injured persons to walk.

Kidney.　A bean-shaped organ (there are two in the body) contained in the urinary tract which filters waste material and fluids not needed by the body.

Kidney stones.　Also known as calculi. They are an accumulation of body salts in the kidney which become hardened masses.

Laminectomy.　An operation sometimes used to relieve pressure on the spinal cord. Also used to examine the extent of damage to cord in special cases.

Lithotripsy.　Procedure for crushing bladder or kidney stones.

Long-legged brace.　Device which supports the leg to aid a person in walking.

Lumbar.　Refers to the vertebrae in the region located between the thoracic vertebrae and sacral vertebrae, or the lower back.

Minipress.　An alpha blocker which is used to relax the urinary sphincter.

Myelogram.　An opaque liquid is injected into the spinal canal that produces an outline of it on X-rays or fluoroscope.

Necrosis.　The death of living tissue.

Neurectomy.　An operation in which the nerves to particular muscles are cut to eliminate severe spasticity in them.

Neurite. Another name for an axon. *See* Axon.

Neurogenic bladder. Refers to the interference in bladder function resulting from a spinal cord injury. Nerve pathways are interrupted which causes an individual to have little or no knowledge of the need to empty the bladder or to prevent the bladder from emptying.

Neuron. Nerve cell.

Occupational therapy. Program designed to teach a person about personal care on activities of daily living (*See* ADL). Activities are used to assist in restoring or improving function. The occupational therapist works very closely with the physical therapist to ensure that an individual reaches his or her highest level of functioning.

Orthosis. A device used to support or brace a weak or disabled joint or muscle (i.e., hand splint, leg brace).

Para. *See* Paraplegic.

Paraparesis. Paralysis of two extremities.

Paraplegia. Occurs when there is injury to the spine at the thoracic or chest level resulting in paralysis of the legs and lower parts of the body.

Paraplegic. Term used for a person who has sustained a spinal injury resulting in paralysis of the lower extremities.

Percutaneous nephrostomy. Procedure in which an instrument is inserted through the skin to remove kidney stones.

pH. Degree of acidity in the urine. High levels of pH contribute to the likelihood of producing urinary stones.

Phenoxybenzamine. Drug used to relax the urethra and aid the process of urination.

Phrenic nerves. Nerves which cause the diaphragm to contract.

Physiatrist. A doctor whose specialty is physical medicine and rehabilitation.

Physical therapy. Program designed to improve remaining physical abilities and to achieve the maximum in activities dependent upon the level of injury (i.e., exercises and activities used to strengthen muscles, increase mobility of the body). *Also see* Occupational therapy.

PNS (peripheral nervous system). Refers to nerves that feed into the central nervous system; includes all nerves in the body except the brain, the spinal cord, and the optic nerves.

Postural drainage. A type of physical therapy in which a person's upper body in tilted in such a way as to clear fluid from the lungs.

Pressure sore/pressure ulcer. *See* Decubitus ulcer.

Prosthesis. A device used as a substitute for a missing part of the body (i.e., artificial leg or arm).

Quad. *See* Quadriplegic.

Quadraparesis. Paralysis of four extremities.

Quadriplegia. Occurs when injury to the spine in the cervical area (neck) causes paralysis in both arms and legs.

Quadriplegic. Term used for a person who has sustained an injury to the spinal cord in the area of the neck causing paralysis in both arms and legs.

Rectal stimulation. Manual stimulation of the rectum to facilitate evacuation of the lower bowel.

Reflex voiding. Occurs when urination is accomplished by a reflex action which tells the body to eliminate urine from the bladder.

Reflux. Urine backs up from the bladder and into the kidneys.

Regeneration. Regrowth of a body or body part. In the spinal cord, it refers to the regrowth of axons (part of nerve cell) after injury.

Residual urine. Refers to urine remaining in the bladder after voiding occurs.

Rhizotomy. An operation to cut certain nerve roots in order to stop severe spasticity.

Robotics. Various types of technology used apart from the individual to perform tasks that otherwise could not be completed by the disabled person (i.e., using a robotic arm for feeding oneself).

Sacral. Pertains to the bottom section of the spinal column or tailbone.

Sacrum. Bone structure in last section of spinal column just above the coccyx.

Schwann cells. *See* Glial cells. A type of glial cell that surrounds peripheral nerves.

Spasm. An involuntary contraction of the muscle or muscles which may interfere with function.

Spasticity. An involuntary jerking of the muscles. These spasms differ from the action of the involuntary muscles of the body in that they occur in those muscles that used to be under the control of the brain before injury.

Sphincter. A circular muscle which contracts or closes a bodily orifice, such as the anus and the bladder.

SSDI (Social Security Disability Insurance). An insurance program administered by the Social Security Administration which provides federal financial assistance to individuals eligible due to a physical or mental disability. It is intended to provide benefits to cover earnings lost resulting from a total disability.

SSI (Supplement Security Income). A financial aid program funded by the federal government. Benefits are based upon a person's physical or mental disability and level of income. Its purpose is to ensure that a person's basic living needs are met.

Suprapubic catheter. A tube which is inserted in the bladder through an opening in the skin in the lower abdomen to allow urine to drain from the bladder.

Suprapubic cystostomy. A small opening made in the bladder in order to remove large stones or establish suprapubic catheter urinary drainage.

Tetraplegia. *See* Quadriplegia.

Texas catheter. *See* Gizmo; external urine collecting device used by males.

Thoracic. Refers to the chest area.

Transection. To cut across. Term generally used to describe the spinal cord being severed or cut.

Trochanter. The upper part of the thighbone.

Urea. A waste product carried out of the body by urination.

Ureter. Tube, of which there are two in the body, which carries urine from the kidneys to the bladder.

Ureterovesical junction. Valve located between the ureter and bladder which keeps urine from backing up from the bladder to the kidneys.

Urethra. Tube which carries urine from the bladder outside the body.

Urodynamics. Studies or tests of the urinary system which provide information relevant to bladder management.

Vertebrae. The bones that make up the spine.

Vocational rehabilitation. Program which assists the individual in matching his or her own physical and mental abilities with types of occupations which may be available.

Wheelchair. A chair equipped with wheels which provides a means of mobility to an individual who is nonambulatory.

Wheelchair cushion. Cushion (of which there are many varieties) which is placed on the seat of a wheelchair to reduce and prevent the problem of pressure sores and biomechanical deformities and to ensure comfort for the wheelchair user.

White matter. One of two major sections of the spinal cord which contains glial cells and axons (*See* Glial cells and Axons).

Appendix 5. Publications

Accent on Living. Accent Publications, P.O. Box 700, Bloomington, IL 61701.

Access Information Bulletin. Paralyzed Veterans of America, 801 18th St., N.W., Washington, DC 20006.

American Rehabilitation. Rehabilitation Services Administration. Order through Superintendent of Documents, U.S. Government Printing Office, Washington, DC 20402.

Careers and the Handicapped. John R. Miller III, publisher, Careers and the Handicapped, 44 Broadway, Greenlawn, NY 11740.

Discover. Time, Inc., 10880 Wilshire Blvd., Los Angeles, CA 90024–4193.

HIMA Focus. Health Industry Manufacturers Association, 1030 Fifteenth St., N.W., Washington, DC 20005–1598.

Homecare. Miramar Publishing Co., 2048 Cother Ave., Los Angeles, CA 90025.

Journal of Rehabilitation Research and Development. Office of Technology Transfer (153D), Publications Circulation Dept., Veterans Administration Medical Center, 50 Irving St., N.W., Washington, DC 20422.

Journal of the American Paraplegia Society. The American Paraplegia Society, 432 Park Ave. South, New York, NY 10016.

Monthly Report. Eastern Paralyzed Veterans Association, 432 Park Ave. South, New York, NY 10016.

Paraplegia News. Paralyzed Veterans of America, 801 Eighteenth St., N.W., Washington, DC 20006.

Rehabilitation Gazette. Edited by G. Laurie and J. Raymond. Gazette International Networking Institute, 4502 Maryland Ave., St. Louis, MO 63108.

Rehabilitation Literature. National Easter Seal Society, 2023 West Ogden Ave., Chicago, IL 60612.

Rehabilitation Report. Hanley & Belfus, Inc., 210 South 13th St., Philadelphia, PA 19107.

Rehabilitation R&D Progress Reports (annual). Office of Technology Transfer (153D), Publications Circulation Dept., Veterans Administration Medical Center, 50 Irving St., N.W., Washington, DC 20422.

Sports 'N Spokes. Paralyzed Veterans of America, 5201 N. 19th Ave., Phoenix, AZ 85015.

Subject Index

Subject Index